# STRUGGLE
## well
# LIVE
### well

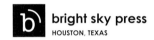
**bright sky press**
HOUSTON, TEXAS

2365 Rice Blvd., Suite 202
Houston, Texas 77005

ISBN: 978-1-942945-42-0

10   9   8   7   6   5   4   3   2   1

Library of Congress Cataloging-in-Publication Data on file with publisher.

Editorial Direction, Lucy Herring Chambers
Managing Editor, Lauren Gow
Cover Design, Jennifer Gilliland
Design, Marla Y. Garcia

Printed in Canada through Friesens

# STRUGGLE well

# LIVE well

## 60 WAYS TO NAVIGATE LIFE'S GOOD, BAD, AND IN-BETWEEN

KEVIN GILLILAND, PSY.D.

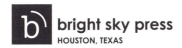

**bright sky press**
HOUSTON, TEXAS

# TABLE OF CONTENTS

# PREFACE
## Struggle Well, Live Well

The title of this book is a cornerstone of my approach to life: my personal life, the lives of my friends, and the lives of my clients.

We'll definitely go through periods of life when we struggle. Some people live under the myth that we can lead a pain-free existence, that we can avoid chapters of struggle. When we start to think that way, our anxiety grows, anticipating the possibility of something painful happening. In order to avoid the other shoe dropping, we'll rob ourselves of joy. That's no way to live.

But when we understand that we'll struggle for chapters in our lives, it somehow makes life a little bit easier. The awareness makes life a little more normal for us. And it also confines the struggle to a smaller chunk of our life.

That's what struggling well is all about, and for quite some time, my mantra was just "struggle well." But conversations with a colleague helped me see things differently.

After we struggle well, we should settle into a time of our lives when we *live well*, when we have meaningful relationships that sustain us, encourage us, challenge us to be better and to take risks. We reach out to people because we know what it's like to struggle. And it's a wonderful feeling to know that our pain and suffering can make someone's burden a little lighter. We can use those times when we're emotionally and physically healthy to step into activities that get us outside and allow us to take risks, learn more about ourselves, and minimize self-criticism.

Living well is about planning for the future, as well as living in the present and enjoying each moment. It's about sitting with friends at dinner and not worrying about tomorrow or the tasks waiting at the office. Living well means we take the time to enjoy a breathtaking mountain or beach view or even a spectacular sunset from our own backyard. It means that we're settled and at peace.

If you find yourself in moments where you should be living well but aren't, then you have some work to do. It doesn't mean you need to see a therapist the rest of your life, although it may be helpful to see someone who has the ability to tell you the truth. It may just mean that you need to get to the bottom of why you haven't been able to find moments in life where you live well.

I know beyond a shadow of a doubt that somebody will read this and think, "You don't know me or the life I've had."

You're right, I don't. But I know many people who have suffered incredible hardships and discovered how to live well *and* struggle well. That's why I know you can do the same. Yes, it takes hard work. But if you're willing to put forth the effort, you'll struggle well and live well in no time.

# INTRODUCTION

**B**efore you start reading this book, there's something you should know about its author: I, Kevin Gilliland, believe the world is flat.

Now, I know there's been some controversy. I know others think differently. But I'm convinced the world is flat, and I don't care what Stephen Hawking has to say about it.

How can I be so sure? After nearly thirty years of working with perfectly rational, intelligent folks who have bank accounts and can spell their names correctly, not a day goes by I don't shake my head at the number of stories I hear about these people sailing right over the edge. Just like the *Niña*, the *Pinta*, and the *Santa María*—clean off the face of the earth!

If you watch people long enough to see what kind of poor decisions we can make, I think you'll come around to my way of seeing things. I think you'll also agree that most people who sail off the edge don't seem to be trying that hard to do it. It just kind of happens.

But here's something else. In all my years as a professional therapist, I couldn't begin to count how many people I know who have avoided the edge and gone on to sail in clear, blue waters. I can also tell you that many of them were able to do so without even trying that hard.

Marital problems, alcohol addiction, sex addiction, anxiety and worry, relationship issues, trauma, grief, body image, depression, dependencies of all kinds—I have seen many people deal head-on with these and other problems and conquer them. I've even seen boats rise up from the edge and get back on course.

Sometimes they needed counseling. Sometimes they needed medication. I'm an advocate of both, but I've also learned that sometimes neither is useful. The truth is that for all the things counseling and medication can do for us, there are countless things they can't do.

The solutions to our problems are often right in front of our bewildered faces. We don't see them because we're too busy listening to friends and family with good intentions give us less than stellar advice. "I don't think they appreciate how hard you work," they say. "You should just quit the job."

This book is about giving you the tools to take back your life in a smart, effective, and proven way. You'll find real answers to real human problems both large and small. And while I believe many of those answers are already rattling around somewhere in our brains, I know that for the majority of us, all it takes is a different perspective or a little nudge to get us back on course. Every once in a while it takes a wise old man walking past to pick the answer up off the ground, dust it off, and say, "Here you go."

And I am not saying that I'm particularly wise, but in counseling men and women with a variety of struggles for three decades, I've learned a thing or two about human nature.

If you're looking for self-help, this is not the book for you. You're going to find that willing yourself to be better, act better, talk better, and look better are not going to work in the long run, which is why you won't find advice like that here. You're also going to find that if you keep buying books to solve problems, you're never going to solve the real problem, which is a self-help book-buying problem. And I'm about solving problems, not encouraging them.

The wisdom in this book is not mumbo-jumbo or metaphysical nonsense that I told Siri® to record on the way to work. This is knowledge I've accumulated from nearly thirty years of working in healthcare. This is knowledge you can put into practice. And I hope that you will give it a try because that's where growth lies.

If you think your problem is more urgent or more serious than the scope of this book, I encourage you to see a professional. Better safe than sorry. But if any of the topics covered in this book have any relation to what it is you're going through, I guarantee you'll find something of great value that you can put into practice immediately.

It might just keep you from sailing over the edge.

# CHAPTER one
# TEACHER

# LIFE IS THE BEST TEACHER

If you're reading this book, you've had a little bit of school. If you are mildly neurotic and went to graduate school, you've had a lot of teachers. But nobody, and I mean nobody, can teach like Life. Be careful what you ask for; she's a brutal teacher.

Her laws are pretty consistent. Sure there are exceptions, but look at the patterns and principles. She is pretty consistent. What drives us mad is when Life switches things up. Learning from Life is about dealing with the curveballs she tosses our way.

Life teaches not only us but our friends and family as well. If we'll just stay out of the way, she'll teach the ones we love some of the most valuable lessons they'll need to function in the world. And by the way, it can be wildly entertaining to watch her teach—downright hilarious at times.

So, if Life is the ultimate teacher, what is our responsibility as parents? One of our roles is to prepare our children for Life. That means our kids are going to suffer and struggle before they get to where they need to be. Our ability to tolerate their suffering and struggling will determine our ability to teach them and to let them learn. It never ceases to amaze me how much we talk about saving for college so our kids can get a "good education." Meanwhile, we have robbed them of learning throughout junior high and high school. If you write letters to your kid's school and coaches or feel the need to explain why they don't get to be on the cheer team or football team, you have robbed your kids of learning. Hang that thought on their participation trophy.

Unless we want our kids living at home when they're thirty-five, with us writing letters to their boss about how they were unjustly fired from the job, it's important to narrow the gap between our teaching as parents and the teaching that Life gives to our kids.

Life really is a caring teacher, and when we quit fighting her rules and guidelines, we start to realize that. I know I did.

# THE EARTH IS FLAT

I still believe the earth is flat, and I've got proof. I get a chance to work with people all the time who are struggling. I also have friends and meet strangers who will, upon hearing what I do, share a struggle that a friend of theirs is having. After hearing endless stories like these, I've come to the conclusion that I have written onto the hard drive of my brain: There is no more powerful force in nature than the human mind bent on a particular course of action.

There are times in our life when we fix our minds on something or someone in an unhealthy way. We do it for a variety of reasons: sometimes it's boredom, other times it's because someone or something is forcing us to wait, think, or be different than we want to be. And we will relentlessly pursue our fixation, even if it means sailing right off the edge of the earth. I kid you not; I just walked out of a session where I saw the stern of the ship disappear over the edge. Disappear!

If you've been in that situation, you know what I'm talking about. It doesn't matter how many colleagues talk to you or how many friends share their wisdom with you. When we're in that situation, it's like we can't hear what anybody has to say. Our sails are up and, in our minds, there's only one logical path to follow—straight over.

It might be an obsession with clothes, houses, people, or any number of things. Regardless of the actual object of our desire, the situation can become tragic when we have a commitment to something but become distracted by something else we believe is better or will fill a hole in our life. That usually means we're not living well with the thoughts and feelings we have about our situation. It almost always means we want to be distracted from the issue at hand.

Whether we are oblivious to our fixations or have an inkling we might be fixated on something, we have to wrap our heads around the idea that maybe we're not fully listening to our friends or that maybe some of what they have to say is valid. When we're constantly discounting, rejecting, or shooting holes in other people's ideas, we need to step back and reassess the situation. Even if we sense they might be speaking the truth, it's difficult for us to overcome our emotions and actually consider what they have to say.

If we can't allow the observations and thoughts of others to come into our decision-making process, then we are at risk of sailing over the edge. We will buy things we regret, end relationships we shouldn't, and quit jobs that are wonderful because we didn't realize that our personal lives were to blame. We made our personal lives unmanageable to the point that we asked the job to fix it for us. No job can ever fix a life.

What should you do if one of your friends is sailing toward the edge of the earth? Be very, very careful. I talk to people and help them for a living. I never get in the way of someone who has full sails and is heading to the edge of the earth. I don't want to get dragged over the edge.

If you think someone isn't listening, it's probably because you're right: they're not listening. So stop saying the same thing over and over: it's not working. Pray hard. Meditate. Hope. Maybe, just maybe, someone will come into their life that they can hear and that speaks their frequency. Say little. But stay in the relationship if at all possible. They are going to need you when they sail off the edge.

# RELEASE THE TRIGGERS IN YOUR LIFE

We all have triggers. It might be your spouse's "mhm" when you tell her you had to work late. It might be your coworker's open discussion of your fashion sense. Maybe stepping on the kids' toys riles you up. Hey, Legos® hurt!

Triggers are just the signals our brain sends us to say, "I have an issue with that." More often than not, our triggers are tiny little things. But when something or somebody pulls them, we go off like a twelve-pound cannon.

We'll even admit, "You know, when you say that, it immediately ruins my day." What we're saying is that there are things that happen in the world that can turn our mood upside down on a dime. That mood change then pushes our behavior in a certain direction. Triggers don't just make us feel differently, they make us act differently, too.

Negative events can trigger a cascade of negative thoughts and emotions. They flash in and out of our brains so fast that it's difficult to process them, much less alter their course or bring them to a halt. Sometimes events trigger our deepest anxieties. "Does my husband really love me? Is he mad at me? Am I terrible parent?" The list goes on.

And because we think in storyboards, our brains start creating stories that, true or not, affect how we feel and act. There's almost always an accompanying thought or series of thoughts or beliefs that we use to fill in the blanks when our moods turn sour. Like, "Oh my gosh, she must be cheating on me," or "I just know they're laughing at that stain on my shirt."

It takes a deep breath, a step back, an analysis of the situation, and a strong commitment to realize that certain events are triggering certain emotions and changes in our behavior. Maintaining an awareness of our triggers and how they affect our thinking is challenging, but if we do it right, we stand a good chance of conquering our emotions and learning to think the best thoughts about a situation before we react.

You need your best thinking. I say it all the time. And that thinking is an active process, not the typical passive process we take. We look at our thoughts like we are watching a movie; we sit there and watch all of this unfold before our eyes in high definition color and Dolby® sound. Our thoughts should be like a conversation or debate with a friend. We should be on our toes, actively challenging things we think are absurd *(because they probably are)*.

One of our greatest weaknesses is that our "thought life" (that world inside our brains that cooks up rational and irrational thoughts alike) gets relegated to this unimportant status, and we can't figure out why we struggle so much.

We've got to put a spotlight on our "thought life" and figure out what kind of changes we need to make to it. That's when we stop doing our worst thinking and start doing our best thinking.

# SEARCH FOR THE TRUTH: FACTS VS FEELINGS

People in my field talk about thoughts, feelings, and behavior all the time. But for some reason, feelings always get the short end of the stick. Why is that?

I think it's because we're not really sure how to manage our feelings, how to look at them, or how to categorize them. And, they're always accompanied by thoughts. They work together. Quite often, we get to our feelings by following the breadcrumbs of thoughts.

Feelings (or we can call them emotions) are unbelievably powerful. They're important components of our daily lives. They are the reason that life has color. And they often seem just as real as any object we can touch.

Again, after lots of conversations, I've written a saying on the hard drive of my brain: Our feelings are true, but they're not *the* truth.

Because they can be so powerful, we often mistake our feelings for the truth. Our feelings are true and authentic, but when we look around, we may realize that our feelings are not grounded in truth. They are shaped by our past experiences, our current expectations, and a host of relationships and thoughts about ourselves.

For example, if we feel threatened by someone, there's no doubt our feelings are authentic. But they may not be justified. Is the person really threatening us? If not, then our feelings are somehow disconnected from the reality of our situation, and that's when we need to step in and try to fix the rift. We have to ask ourselves: Do I feel like this in similar situations? What is the emotion I am actually feeling?

What are the thoughts I'm having? Would other people feel this way? Who does this person remind me of? Are my thoughts reasonable or catastrophic? What's the evidence to support my feelings?

If we're feeling sad, let's take a look around and see if our feelings correspond with our situation. We may find that our situation is pretty good—decent buddies, decent house, decent car—but the sadness just doesn't go away. There's probably something else going on, something deeper, and our feelings are trying to tell us that.

In his book *Blink*, Malcolm Gladwell talks about this uncanny ability we have to make decisions and come to conclusions in the blink of an eye. We're not really sure how this happens. But it involves feelings, as if we can sense through intuition what the best path forward will be.

So, feelings can sometimes come very close to facts. We've got to take them seriously, not toss them to the side just because they can be difficult to handle or to define.

At the same time, feelings carry a natural subjectivity with them, so we have to be careful about what we do with them. We should hold on loosely to our feelings to ensure we are receptive to them but not slaves to them, because feelings do not always represent the truth.

# THOUGHTS MATTER, THE SPACE IS REAL

At some point in our life we start to realize how active our minds are and how often we rehearse conversations or events before we act. At least a lot of us do. We often talk about it happening in a split second, as if there is no space between the thought and the action or the flood of emotion. It may feel that way, but in most cases, it's not that way. And it's in that space that we have a chance for a very different experience. A very different life.

The space exists; it's real. As real as anything in this world that you can touch. But if we don't look for it, if we don't strive for it, we may end up living a life of impulse and chasing after the wind without the faintest idea why.

We see the consequences of ignoring the space in every aspect of life. Obesity, addiction, pornography, debt—the list is endless. The problem begins to surface when we realize that a lot of our thoughts, the majority for some people, can be quite negative and critical. It's not very often I meet someone who has a thought life that is naturally positive and encouraging. When we struggle, there is almost always a stream of incredibly negative thoughts. If you listen, you will hear professionals—even athletes and entertainers, and yes, therapists—talk about this.

The more I work with people when they are struggling, the more I have become aware of the struggles we face when we're not active in our thinking. The problem is that we are *always* thinking, but not necessarily in an active, participatory way. The other day, I heard the statement, "We can't hide from our thoughts." I love that because, in a way, it's true.

We allow negative thoughts to take up every square inch of our mind, and we do nothing to throw them out like the garbage they are. They're the kind of thoughts that are based on nothing, that do nothing for us, and that we allow to run around in our heads without a leash as if they're having no negative effects on us.

I've counseled dozens of divorced people who have this mistaken idea that all of the terrible, hurtful things their ex-husbands or ex-wives said about them had no effect on them because they were divorced. Nothing could be further from the truth. We don't need those kinds of thoughts in our database. They are not neutral. They take a toll on us.

We need to be active and guarded with our mind and how it works. We need to realize that one of the greatest gifts is the opportunity that opens up in the space between the stimulus and the response. That space allows us to choose a different path. One of the most commonly travelled bad paths is to act as though we can tell the future, predict what is going to happen *(and it's usually a bad outcome we forsee)*. If we can step back and realize that we really aren't as good at predicting the future as it seems, and instead make a decision to wait on the worry, we have a chance to struggle less. We can live this day, with all its challenges, and manage tomorrow when it gets here. We don't need to borrow trouble from tomorrow, especially when we don't know if it's going to show up.

It's simple. Slow down. Take some time before you respond to a stimulus. And, please, know the difference between real and imagined. And expand your list of possibilities, your list of options. When in doubt, choose an option that may be a little more reasonable, a little more fair. Our thoughts tend toward catastrophe; they are rarely fair. If you can, choose an option you would say to a friend if they were in your situation. It's not easy. I said it was simple, I didn't say easy.

We need our best thinking. Being more aware and involved with what goes on inside our heads is a good place to start. A great place actually.

# BREAK IT UP

We break our lives down into chunks for a reason. We break miles into feet, food into portions, and big projects into phases. If we borrowed from the same playbook when it came to eating healthier, drinking less, parenting better, spending time with friends and family, or learning to play guitar, we might even achieve those goals and enjoy the journey.

Perhaps we're trying to change our outlook on life. Or, we just want our days to be brighter. Whatever type of change we want to make, here's something that might make it a little more manageable: break it up.

We all have days and sometimes weeks when we have a million things to do, pressure at the office, challenges with kids, and the feeling that you just can't get it all done or that things will never get better. Break up the day and the routine. We should pick a morning to just sit quietly, reflect, or read a book. After thinking about all of the great things that are happening in our lives, we'll go on about our day just a little differently. No, it won't fix everything; it can't, and we shouldn't expect it to. However, setting aside a quiet, contemplative time without the distractions might give us a manageable path to a happier, more optimistic us. And all it took was a single step forward.

Or, maybe we're trying to cut back on our alcohol intake. We pick a night and commit to not drinking that evening. Conscious, small-scale decisions like that set the tone for achieving big things and for making healthy changes in our lifestyle. Once we have conquered one night's drinking, another night's is within our reach. Success can be contagious.

For those struggling with depression, waking up each morning sometimes feels like we've got this fog hanging over us. It's typical to think, "I don't feel like calling a friend or hanging out with somebody today. I don't even feel like getting out of bed." I get it. But still, just call one friend. Not every day. Not a dozen friends. Just one. Just today. If we call them, there's a decent chance that just hearing their voice will make us want to get lunch or see a movie with them.

## Life gets a lot simpler and easier when we break it down into small steps.

I don't care who we are or what we're trying to do. Make it easier. Be smart. Learn from the other places in life where we see people accomplish all manner of amazing things; one bite, one step, one stroke, one letter, one question, or one note at a time. We don't have to swallow the whole enchilada at once.

On our way to the top, it's important to remember how others have made the journey. Giant leaps will never get us there. Only consistent, manageable steps in the right direction can get us where we need to go.

# CHANGE: THE KEY INGREDIENT

If drinking Diet Coke® was an Olympic sport, my wife would be a world record holder. That is until she got pregnant and stopped downing the stuff altogether.

I was so impressed by her willpower. And being the sensitive husband that I am, I asked her (with a Diet Coke in my hand, of course), "Why did you quit?"

"Because the doctor said drinking them isn't good while you're pregnant," she responded. I was just amazed at her determination.

I kid you not, within an hour of giving birth, she pulled me in by the collar and said, "Where's my Diet Coke?" True story.

That was the day I learned there is a big difference between compliance and change. It turns out that we have a knack for compliance. We can eat healthy or exercise consistently when someone is with us or watching us.

One of the unique qualities most humans share is the deeply-rooted desire to improve, to get better at something, to transform an area of their lives. Whether that's related to work, relationships, or health, we recognize that there are some things we need to stop doing and some things we want to start doing. Acknowledging this concept and the moment when it happens in our lives is one of the key ingredients that allow us to grow and mature.

It's only taken me about twenty years to get that idea settled into my life. It's rather embarrassing to admit what I originally thought about change when I started working with people. I actually thought that if someone took the time out of a busy schedule and paid me to talk about things that were very difficult, then that person must be ready to change. I began to realize over time that scheduling a meeting with a therapist actually told me very little about the desire to change, the motivation to change, or even any belief about the possibility of change. And that's what the research says, not just my impressions. (Didn't know that before I spent five years in graduate school.)

I've learned from therapy and research that we need to start the process of change where we *are*, not where we think we *should* be. Take, for instance, New Year's resolutions. A lot of people think they need to get healthy in the New Year, probably because of excessive eating and lack of exercise during the holidays. So, every health club in the month of January is packed. But most of the newcomers at the gym don't really want to change; they just feel bad about the choices made over the past couple of weeks. Rather than over-committing, it would be better if they start walking or jogging a couple of times a week.

There is a difference between compliance and change. Compliance is usually done for someone else, their idea, request, or order. It's somebody trying to change us. I often say, "I'm not sure where in the city my wife is right now, but if she's talking to a friend about something she thinks I need to change, I can feel that conversation twenty miles away, and I'll start my resistance."

People hate being changed. Compliance is just a strategy people use to get others to quit talking to them about what they ought to do. But if I'm actually open to change, if I'm the one doing the work, then I just might end up starting a change process that lasts. For that to occur, there has to be something that happens internally as well as externally.

Even though we know deep down that change can be a positive thing, it's still both fascinating and mysterious to not only observe the process in others, but to also experience it firsthand. If you're willing to take the risk of changing, then you will never be, as Teddy Roosevelt once said, "A cold and timid soul that knows neither victory nor defeat."

# IT'S HARD TO BE A NEW PERSON IN AN OLD PLACE

I work with people daily who have a deep, sincere, personal desire and commitment to make healthy changes. They've come to see me because they don't like what is happening in their lives—whether their situation involves the way they use alcohol, pain meds, food, or because their marriage isn't working.

They are motivated and hard-working individuals. Yet when they step into their lives with new insight and a plan to change, they realize how difficult it is to be a new person in an old place.

It is fascinating how their "old" world sometimes greets them.

We all live in a way that people expect certain things from us, good and bad, because over time our personality becomes part of other peoples' lives. They know us.

When we change something significant about ourselves (let's say, for example, our intake of alcohol), a massive shift in thinking and feeling occurs internally. Externally, our friends and family might know only the tip of our iceberg, even when we might have shared openly about what we want to change about ourselves. However, most don't understand the full extent of our hopes, fears, dreams, sleepless nights, and regrets that can haunt us while we wrestle with our issue.

The struggle, then, becomes translating our newfound insight into behaviors. Insight without behavioral change leaves everybody feeling a little disappointed. What we ultimately want is for the changes we desire to inhabit our "new" world.

Let's not be naïve about this transformation. Expect the journey to be surprising and challenging. That's why we need to be smart about moving forward. The fact is that humans seeking to change do better when they're around other people. We just do better in groups—regardless of whether we're a "people person" or not. Groups allow us to see different perspectives; group members can challenge us in indirect ways; we can hear different approaches; and we can think differently about our situations. Because relationships provide encouragement, they can give us hope when our commitment begins to lag. Groups help us keep the momentum going.

Sometimes, we have to do things (like joining a support group or reaching out to a friend) that give us new information we can use to think differently about our situation. We must act our way into thinking differently. When those valuable moments occur, when our new thoughts lead to a new discovery—well, the momentum becomes a movement. That's when new overtakes old, and we're on our way to a better life.

# CHAPTER

## two

# RELATIONSHIPS

# IDENTITY: FINDING AND FANNING THE FLAMES OF WHO WE REALLY ARE

These days, families come in all shapes and sizes. Whether we admit it or not, we all take on very distinct roles within our families. The entertainer, the smart one, the responsible one, the hero—the list is long. When we reach adulthood and step outside of this small world, we may struggle to figure out who we really are and what the heck we're supposed to be doing with our life.

We all have talents and a specific set of strengths. These span from the obvious (singing, dancing, academic proficiency, athletic ability, etc.) to the subtle (problem-solving, interpersonal relationships, intuitive thinking, emotional intelligence, etc.). But how we see these talents—and whether we act on them at all—is often clouded by the roles we played in our early years and the expectations of others.

One of the most important outlets for identity is the career we choose. Sometimes we fall into the trap of choosing something we like rather than something we're really good at. Other times, we select a job based on what we think our spouse or parents want.

Maybe we come from a long line of lawyers, and we grew up with the looming legacy of our father and his father and his father and their heavy expectations for us to follow suit. Or maybe we were raised by parents who couldn't afford to go to college and saved their whole lives to send us to college so we could make a good living, so we'd better ditch those plans to be an artist and study to become a doctor.

The problem with making choices this way is that our life isn't about us anymore. It's about everyone else. And the worst part is that we don't always realize that it's happening. Those old family roles can be a silent powerful undercurrent, pulling us from where we're really meant to be. And while this kind of pressure may seem outdated and absurd, you'd be shocked at how often I hear this from college students and their parents.

Some parents are very subtle and absolutely don't see that they are directing their child's career, but just ask their young adult when the parents aren't around and watch their reaction. Yeah, they feel it and know it. And they hate it.

Living someone else's life is very difficult. People can do it for a while, and some settle into it and even learn to like it—like an arranged marriage. But for many, it catches up with them. It can be a confusing time for people who *thought* what their parents wanted was what they wanted. They just don't realize they never had a chance to give input or have a vote. If we feel trapped, we usually open ourselves up to all manner of craziness. We know the list: depression, alcohol, pornography, food—the usual suspects that take our minds off the misery we live in day after day.

But no matter where we are in life, it's never too late to change directions.
We need to live a life that fits who we really are. Yes, even if we have kids and a mortgage. Sure, it may take a little more planning and a gentle transition. But try it. Pursuing something we excel at and love energizes us, whether that means a complete career switch to a new "second act" or dusting off your art supplies on the weekend. If you fan the flames of who you really are, I guarantee you won't regret it.

# THE BIRD DIDN'T SH*T ON YOU

I'm not going to name names because that would be rude. But, we all know that there are times when our perspective warps our life.

One of the times when we tend to have high expectations is when we host an event, dinner, gathering, or party. We exhaust ourselves trying to achieve a level of perfection and excellence, trying to think of everything. That may not be a realistic goal. We become aware of our expectations when we start to watch how people react, or don't react, to the things we hoped they would like, enjoy, or be surprised by when we planned the thing weeks ago. Here's the truth: people's reactions may have absolutely nothing to do with you or what you've done to prepare for that event.

Let's consider the example of a typical bird—carefree, flying, going about his day. Here you come, on a mission to get somewhere on time and looking good, when all of a sudden . . . Holy crap! He got you.

Really? You think that bird picked you out for this honor? No, no. It didn't. That isn't how the bird works. Yet, you take it personally—as though the bird had *you* in his sights.

When it comes to how things work in our lives, you must know by now that people show up with their own baggage, and it's full of emotions, expectations, and behaviors.

Their bag of issues most likely will have nothing to do with you, but when we see the bag being slung around, we do what so many others do: we believe (if not say), "When I see you do that, the story I make up in my head is that I am to blame; I'm an idiot; I'm a worthless, blah, blah, blah..." Our minds quickly fill with thoughts, and they are almost always fast and negative.

We personalize other people's issues when they bring them into our world or gatherings. And when we do that, we are taking a step down a bad path. We create an opening for resentment, anger, and misinterpretation of very basic information and interactions. We start making emotional and irrational decisions. It takes us off our game, and we are never good when that happens. Life is challenging; we need our best game.

The next time someone brings baggage into your life, catch yourself before you respond. Sometimes we need to let their behavior pass right on by and pay it no attention. Other times we need to examine the thoughts running through our heads and get busy. Start challenging the thoughts. Are they accurate? Are they true? Are they valid? Are they catastrophic? But whatever you do, don't let them run free in your head; they will take up every square inch of space. And when our heads are crowded with negative thoughts, it's no wonder we react the way we do.

So, when you see the bird doing its business—at your party or somebody else's—remember this: The bird didn't shit on you, the bird just shit. It's not personal. It's what birds do.

# IT'S NOT WHO YOU PICK

Really, it's not who you pick.

Granted, there are a lot of bad shows on TV. But one of the worst is about how to pick "the right person" for marriage. Let me save you some time. Picking the "the right person" is a myth. I hear people say "she/he is not who I married." And most of the time I think "No. And neither are you."

Here's the assumption: *if I scour my community in the city and possibly even date across the country, I will find my perfect match. And if I find my perfect match, I will stay married and happy the rest of my days.* Seriously, there's no way you can read that with a straight face. But that's what TV wants us to believe, and a lot of us step into marriage believing just that.

It's not who we pick, it's who we become. And when you're in a marriage, you will never be closer to another individual than your spouse. That means you have a tremendous opportunity to experience joys and happiness that you won't find in other areas of your life. It also means you will experience a level of suffering and hardship you wouldn't otherwise experience.

Think about any roommate you've had. You get to know your roommate really well when you're in college or shortly after college. How long does it take for their little habits and behaviors to start to get under your skin? Okay, now imagine living with them the rest of your life. That's marriage. And at the most fundamental level, we have to get past this hurdle before we even get to the meaningful parts of a marriage. If you can't be a good roommate, you don't have a chance of being a good husband or wife.

Marriage is one of the most difficult things we will try to accomplish. It takes work. It takes commitment. The person you pick isn't a perfect person, and neither are you. Remember that. Focusing on who we picked can distract us from the real issue, who are we becoming?

# EIGHTY-SEVEN PERCENT

"**M**y wife is eighty-seven percent." That statement shocked me because it came from a therapist I really admire; I love this guy—he's my favorite curmudgeon. But he could tell from my expression that I was wondering if he ever shared that with his bride.

"Yes! You heard me right," he said. "No matter how hard I try, getting to one hundred percent is impossible." And that's one of the most valuable lessons we can learn in marriage. There's simply no one-hundred-percenter out there for any of us. That's a fact.

We had that discussion at least four or five years ago and have had countless similar ones since. I've come to believe that his statement captures one of the most fundamental truths in marital happiness and offers up the best advice for anyone thinking about getting married.

And taking this as a truth, I have a choice (key word: *choice*). Do I want to focus on the eighty-seven percent or the thirteen percent?

I see quite a few of people chipping away at that thirteen percent; trying to push their partner's number up to ninety-eight percent. That's one strategy. And you know what, we can change, a little bit.

But here's a better strategy: focus on the eighty-seven percent. The eighty-seven percent is always spectacular. Do you know how fortunate you are? It doesn't matter who you're married to, you're never going to make it to one hundred percent. Couples burn a lot of relationship capital and emotional energy trying to get to one hundred percent or ninety-eight percent or ninety-five percent, rather than enjoying the percentage they have.

It's really just about our perspective. It's about perceptions. It's about a choice. Those are concepts I think we all hear about when we step into marriage, but I don't think anything has helped me use these concepts in my marriage more than thinking about that eighty-seven percent.

When we burn all of our resources on a small amount of change rather than enjoying the large percentage of what we already have, we run the risk of destroying our marriage in pursuit of a myth.

Now if that doesn't make you think differently about your marriage, I don't know what will. It makes me wonder what percentage my wife would say I am.

# TOXIC FAMILY MEMBERS

One of the hardest things we face growing up is the fact that our parents are just like the other adults in our life and come with their own unique personalities, quirks, gifts, pains, and suffering.

It's an odd realization that sometimes comes as a bump in the road and sometimes as a giant pothole.

As a young child, your parents are your gateway to the world. And even in your teen years, in the gaps of time when you could admit that you weren't living with the Biggest Idiots on the Planet, you probably looked to them for guidance because you trusted their years of wisdom and experience.

But then it started to occur to you that they aren't always right.

It's a strange thing to accept, but your parents are capable of making mistakes, big and small.

They're human. They get angry and petty. They have foibles and faults. They will sometimes fall short. They're not infallible; and, in some ways, that's a relief. We realize that they struggle and are just as imperfect as we are.

But sometimes, parents can also be cruel. They can be abusive. Some of them struggle with addictions, anxiety, and depression. Some of them abandon the role of parenting, leaving those kinds of things in the hands of their kids.

If we're unfortunate enough to have parents like these, it's not always a simple task to cut them out of our lives, because we can't always tell that we're being poisoned.

We're so tightly bound to our parents that, even if they're toxic, it goes against the core of our nature to cut ties. The same goes for siblings.

I often hear people say that their family issues are "complicated." Usually, they're not. But family is extremely *emotional*. And even if we know that a parent or sibling is doing something harmful to themselves or us, there's often a tendency to defend or deny. Or to take up the slack they have left.

In a way, it feels like a betrayal if we admit it.

Whether we find ourselves dealing with a toxic parent or sibling, stepping away from that relationship doesn't have to be permanent. We might just need to take a break for a while. If you're married, odds are that your spouse has been trying to help you see this for years. Maybe it's time to listen a little more closely to what they have to say. We sometimes just need to get some fresh air. Think of it as a chapter, not the story of a lifetime.

It's not our job to fix them, and it's not our job to alter their negative behaviors. If you try to save a drowning person, you run the risk of going down in their panic.

Instead of having one drowning person, now you have two.

# NO WAY IN HELL I'D GO BACK TO THE TEENAGE YEARS

I believe one of the most important words in any language is "remember." Think about that for a minute. Forgot your anniversary? Bad thing. Remembered your anniversary? Good thing! Forgot where you put your car keys? Bad thing. Remembered where you put your car keys? Good thing!

Forgot what it's like to be a teenager? Bad thing! Face it, most of us are far removed from our teenage years. And I venture a guess that few of us would go back to that stressful, acne-complexion-voice-changing-hormonal-roller-coaster time in our lives. Man, I wouldn't take a million bucks to go through that phase of my life again.

But, as parents or guardians of teenagers, we owe it to our teenager to try and remember just how challenging it was, because that'll give us a really healthy dose of empathy. You know, empathy—that ability to understand and share the *feelings* of others.

Teenagers aren't doing a lot of thinking when their hormones are on a scavenger hunt for normalcy. They are, however, doing a lot of *feeling*. They are volatile, emotional creatures—just like we were—and we should remember (there's that word again) that their feelings are genuine. Maybe their actions could use a little help. But their feelings are raw and powerful and confusing. And that's where we have to connect.

I've seen so many parent-child relationships turn into a hot mess during the teenage years because parents tend to step in with a logical approach to an emotional teenager. All of that can be corrected if we take a step back when our teenager does something stupid and connect with them on an emotional level.

When people know they have been heard and understood, they are more open to discuss different approaches to life. Teenagers are no different. Well, they are, but they are more open to conversations when they know we understand what they are going through.

You didn't do drugs when you were a kid? Good for you! But your teenager just did. And your reaction today could determine your relationship with your teenager forever.

So the next time your teenager makes a bad choice (it will happen), *remember* what it's like to *feel* like a teenager. Remember that it's not easy to be teased. Remember that your emotions were always on high alert. Remember that digital media has forever changed how our kids behave and communicate. Remember that this is just a chapter of their life.

# LONG-TERM RELATIONSHIPS

"**W**hy doesn't my husband (or wife) love me anymore? Where did all of the passion go? Did it fizzle out?"

It's something most married couples eventually ask. They want to know what happened to the spark that first lit their eternal fire. They ask big, sweeping questions, when in reality the answers are usually found in little things.

It's as if one day, they look over at the face that's been their decades-long companion and realize, *My God, you've gotten old/boring/cold/out of shape. When did that happen?* And it's a feeling that sort of makes sense. If you were to eat oatmeal for breakfast every single day for twenty years, there would inevitably come a moment where you dump the porridge down the drain and say, "You know something? I am sick of oatmeal."

You deserve something better than this boring, bland meal, right?

Our brains are designed to respond to various stimuli, and if there's one thing that humans *love*, it's to be stimulated. Yes, these are generalities, but it's hard to dispute that men typically want something novel and interesting put in front of them—something shiny to look at or another spot of light to chase. Women want to feel loved, valued, and connected.

When you and your spouse first started dating, the sparks were flying and stimuli were easy to come by. Everything was new. But over time we settle in, get comfortable, and a little bit lazy. When things feel *blah*, we tend to look at the person across the couch and start to wonder what happened to them.

But if you're feeling like the sizzle is slipping out of your relationship, the first place to start is usually with ourselves. It's such a better place to start for many reasons. First, you have the most control over your behavior (it's hard to change someone else), it has an impact on other people, and it's a gentle way to start a new conversation that may be difficult. It lends a little credibility to your statements when you have been doing something yourself.

Are *you* the one who has gotten old/boring/cold/out of shape? Because somewhere along the way, you may have lost track of yourself—just as you've lost track of your spouse.

So give yourself and your habits a once-over. When was the last time you got a haircut or bought a flattering new outfit? Do you maybe have a few extra pounds around your waist? What was the last spontaneous thing you did? How often do you send a short, loving text or pick up a bouquet of flowers "just because?" We underestimate the power of paying just a bit more attention to our appearance and routinely making a few simple, kind gestures. Yes, it matters. It did when you were dating, and it is probably more important ten or twenty years into the marriage than it was while dating.

And if your partner *has* put on a few pounds, instead of telling them, "Hey, you've gotten kinda fat," why don't you suggest the two of you start walking together or cooking healthy meals? I guarantee you it will be a much more pleasant conversation.

Plus, engaging in shared activities is a proven way to reconnect and *stay connected*. You don't have to take up tandem skydiving; just find something new and jump into it together. Whatever it is, if you're doing something novel and rewarding, your brain will be flooded with mood-boosting chemicals. Remember those from when you started dating?

Being in a long-term relationship with someone is one of the hardest things you'll ever do. But a successful—and even passionate—partnership is possible if you keep putting a little bit of fuel on that fire every day.

# CHAPTER
## three
# GOD

# MAKE YOUR SPIRITUALITY MATTER

Just to be upfront, I am both spiritual and religious. Whether it's in my personal life or at work, I love talking with people about the things that matter, like family, work, and hobbies. Spirituality also happens to be one of those key areas. Religion, too.

But first, let's define the two. Religion is a shared system of beliefs we subscribe to that helps us make sense out of our world. It's a worldview. There are lots of worldviews, like Christianity, Judaism, Buddhism, and Hinduism, to name a few. For some, science is a worldview.

Spirituality, on the other hand, is the application of religion. It's how much (or little) you implement your preferred religious system into your everyday life.

The spiritual side of our lives is unbelievably important because it challenges us to act in ways that are consistent with our religious affiliation.

Sometimes we don't claim our religion because we know that just the mention of a specific religion can quickly turn into a lightning rod for emotions. Bringing up religion can spark heated debates or arguments at any time, in any place, with anybody. So, we generally keep it to ourselves.

To avoid confrontation, we use a more socially acceptable term: we say that we're "spiritual." We can tell people we're spiritual because then we've covered the whole range of religious and even non-religious affiliations. One drawback to the term spiritual is that we usually have no idea what someone means by the term. That can be a good thing if that's what is intended, but it can also leave people wondering.

Religion has been around since the beginning of time, and it's just as important to us today as it was to the ancient Egyptians. History simply does not support the idea that religion is dead or that our need for religious fulfillment is no longer fundamental to who we are.

Take a look at those big stone statues on Easter Island. You think they're just statues? Just some Stone Age adolescent art project?

I'm sure the builders were thinking, "You know what we need? We need some art. We need some big statues of things that have absolutely no religious significance tied to them. Yeah, people are gonna die to haul these massive stone artworks across the continent, but that's just the price of art these days."

No way! The only people who work that hard for something as impossible as that are people with deep, religious motivations. At a time when survival was paramount and hydraulic machines were not even fantasies, it took a people driven by a shared system of beliefs to do something so monumental.

Religion connects us with meaning and purpose. It's part of our DNA. The folks on Easter Island didn't cling to religion just because it was something to do. They sensed a need for meaning. They sought purpose beyond birth, toil, and death.

Spirituality is that wonderful place where our religious beliefs become actionable. Where we put the natural man behind us and seek the guidance and direction of something that's bigger than us and necessary to become a new person.

Spirituality is not a behavioral guide. It doesn't contain a value system that sustains us and keeps us on a particular path.

That's why I'm not that interested in spirituality without religion. Spirituality makes for wonderful dinner conversation, but when it comes time to do the hard work of waking up every morning at 6:00 am, a pristine spirituality without a religious anchoring is going to be of no use to you.

Spirituality has become the cotton candy of religion. Like all cotton candy, it's fluffy and melts on your tongue, but it never satisfies for very long. It only takes a few bites before you realize that what you're eating has no substance, no nutritional value, and is only going to leave you craving a big bowl of french fries.

If you're anchored and doing great in your spiritual life, awesome. If you haven't gotten near anything religious in a while, you may want to rethink that decision. Yes, many of us have been hurt by religion. But we've all been hurt by a lot of things, and we figure out a way to work through it. I've been in a terrible car wreck but I keep driving. It's worth it.

Don't let me turn you off to spirituality. It really can be a beautiful thing. But if you've got nothing substantial to prop it up, then all you've got is a stick of sugar in your hand and a huge cavity waiting to be filled.

# RE-THINKING SPIRITUALITY WITH GOD IN MIND

Much has been written about the "spike in spirituality" that followed the terrorist attacks of September 11, 2001. We heard stories of individuals of all different backgrounds turning to faith and prayer to make sense of the tragedy. We heard prominent religious leaders console a grieving and fearful nation. But as the pain of the tragedy ebbed away, so did the spiritual expression.

It's funny how we look at the notion of God, spirits, and all things eternal in the twenty-first century. It's hard for us as westerners to entertain something that can't be explained or quantified, yet nine in ten Americans consistently claim to believe in God or a higher power, according to a 2015 Pew Research poll.

Not all of us go to church or synagogue or whatever coincides with the faith we hold, but it would be silly to think that the vast majority of Americans do not possess a single ounce of spirituality. We don't often see it or acknowledge it, because spirituality is usually expressed only in times of need, confusion, or hardship.

In the aftermath of 9/11 (or other tragedies), spirituality was not such a sensitive subject. In fact, it was invited into our homes, into newsrooms, and into government spaces. But we've cycled back around, back to normalcy, where spiritual conversations are generally confined to those who share the same faith.

I get it; nobody wants to offend or start an argument. But our spirituality is such a critical element of our humanity. Beyond daily activities, such as eating, sleeping, playing sports, going to work, and hanging with friends, our minds can't help but turn to the bigger picture and explore how we as individuals fit into it. We want solid answers to life's greatest questions. What we don't want are answers that end in "pointlessness" or "hopelessness" or "six weeks to live."

There's a hole in all of us, and to not talk about it or try to fill it with substitutes isn't going to work. We've got to admit there's a hole before we can do anything about it.

And it's not just a twenty-first century problem. Philosophers, theologians, geniuses, and everyday folks have been wrestling about eternity for an eternity. We didn't just start questioning our existence or the meaning of tragic events as soon as the planes hit; we've been doing it for a very long time.

Spiritual expression, while important during trying times, has to outlast the tragedy and continue into normalcy. The void in our souls doesn't get patched up after a prayer and a cappuccino. Just like the eternal nature of our questions, filling that hole is a never-ending task.

The good news is that filling the spiritual void is the only thing that really lasts. We can get those cheap highs, whether it's Friday night margaritas or buying a new car, but I guarantee you from personal experience that cheap highs don't last. Real, lasting fulfillment is a spiritual matter.

STRUGGLE WELL, LIVE WELL

# MEDITATION

**M**editation helps ease one of the key symptoms of anxiety and depression: an overcrowded mind. When we're suffering from anxiety or depression, our minds often become hyper-vigilant, hyperactive, or very selective and biased—meaning depressed, negative, and hopeless.

One of the key elements of treating illnesses like anxiety and depression, which we have learned about from decades of good treatment and research, is to help people be more active in how their mind selects and focuses on certain information. For example, people who are anxious see and look for fearful, harmful things. People who are depressed see sad, negative things. But the reality is that often life is a mixture. It has harmful things, but it has good and safe things, too.

Therapeutic research has shown positive results when we choose to be more active, intentional, realistic, and controlling with the negative things we see or experience. Meditation is a great place to practice having an active mind, to develop a greater sense of control over our thoughts, and to appreciate how those thoughts impact behaviors.

Meditating gets your mind in shape, just like exercising does with any other body part. While it takes time and patience, meditating in small increments begins to foster a healthy routine and gives you new ways of viewing life and its challenges.

Meditation helps with positivity because it involves recognizing the need for gratitude and thankfulness. It causes our minds to focus on the good just as much as the bad. With anxiety and depression, our minds become selective and biased in a negative way. Meditation allows for a fairer assessment of life.

Meditation also helps by orienting us to a more hopeful and optimistic view of the world. It helps us be mindful of a world beyond our own circumstances or struggles. When we're in tune not only with ourselves but also with the needs and hopes of others, we take an important step in a healing process that only meditation can provide.

# MONEY IS NOT THE ROOT OF THE PROBLEM

Repeat after me: *Money is not the problem.*

I think about money like I think about alcohol. Our problem is not alcohol. We tried as a country to ban it, and look where that got us. We're talking speakeasies (love that word) and Al Capone—not exactly America's most wholesome moment.

We ended up teaching ourselves a valuable lesson: people are the real problem. But we can't ban people, now can we?

When it comes to money, something we definitely can't ban, we have to understand that money isn't the source of our problems. It's what we bring to money and what we ask money to do for us that gets us into trouble.

I talk to a lot of financially successful people who struggle with this very issue. They're able to substitute money for things that they actually need to do themselves. In other words, their problems persist because now they pay someone to do things for them. And when they get into trouble, money can get them out of trouble in a snap.

Up to a certain point, money can rescue us.

But just like the people who have an addiction to alcohol or drugs, people who are obsessed with money or with pursuing money have a similar problem on their hands. They can't quit thinking about money and what money can do for them. Like the normal use of alcohol, money is often managed well by people. And like alcohol, in subtle ways it can begin to turn into something very different. We need more and more to get the same feeling.

It's the same with our money problems. We're no longer making money to improve our lives; instead we're measuring how much money we've got today to make sure we'll have more of it if we measure again tomorrow. We sail toward the edge when we begin to ask money to do something for us—bring us happiness, cure our boredom, or relieve the anxiety to provide for family.

Instead, let's focus on the things that we know have far more value than money, like our family or our wellbeing. Take a few moments, maybe even do that meditation thing we talked about earlier, and come back to the things that mattered most to us when life was simpler, slower, and clearer.

And maybe, just maybe, money and how we use it will begin to change.

# DIGNITY IS PART OF YOUR DNA

Do you believe humans are wonderfully made? Do you believe there is something truly inspiring about what the human spirit can do? These are worldviews that are usually tucked into our religious views. You could even say our religious view is our worldview.

What religion tells us is that people are born with a kind of dignity. Of course, being the imperfect humans we are, we don't always recognize or respect that dignity or stop ourselves from violating that dignity.

We don't always respect this innate quality because we often keep our religion and our worldview separate. Some don't even know they're doing it.

It's not unusual to come across church-going or synagogue- and mosque-attending individuals who seem to have two separate lives. Not with all their beliefs, not usually; it's typically a few key beliefs or principles that don't get translated into everyday life. If you say you believe there is this inherent value within every person, then why do you treat the waiter that way or why do you treat the people in your office that way? There's going to be tension in your life and in your soul when you realize that some of your deeply held religious beliefs have not been carrying over into the way you live and treat others.

If you feel it's important to help those who are poor, those who are homeless, or those who are widows and widowers, but you don't give any time or money toward helping them, then your religion is fairly thin. Or, you may not actually value those beliefs after all. You may just think you are supposed to value that. That's just the truth.

If, on the other hand, you devote time and resources to the needy and to those less fortunate than you, then your life is probably pretty well aligned with your religious beliefs. We do better when we live this way. Now, I'm not sure we can actually care about all the things there are to care about in this world. So be honest with yourself; speak and live out the things that matter to you. Leave the rest for other people.

We're fortunate, in some seasons of our life, to have the things we have and to do the things we do. The fact of the matter is that others may be in a chapter that is less fortunate, but no less worthy of being treated with dignity.

If you don't find yourself walking in the path that you talk about, you may need to spend some time getting your words and your works lined up. They should be. Figure out what needs to shift and enjoy the blessing of that path. It's yours.

# WANT TO FEEL BETTER? SERVE OTHERS

I love this quote by British author C.S. Lewis: "Do not waste time bothering whether you 'love' your neighbor; act as if you did."

We think in such limited terms when it comes to treating depression and anxiety. Sure, see a therapist, take your meds, but you know what? Maybe you just need to get outside of your own life and be thoughtful of other people.

One of the most painful symptoms of emotional and physical struggles is isolation. It's also a very common way of coping for people to withdraw when we're struggling. As a result, people pull out of our lives. As we become more disconnected from people, we turn inward and ruminate on our condition, often making our suffering greater.

When we muster the energy to reach out to someone, we discover one of life's great secrets. No matter where you are in life, when you step out of your own world and into someone else's, it changes you. Becoming mindful of other people's struggles helps us live well when we struggle. No, I'm not talking about "misery loves company." Quite the opposite.

I'm talking about serving others, one of the single most effective means by which we can change our outlook on life and change our lifestyle itself. Helping others quiets the noise that suffering generates, and it gives us perspective. It can also give us hope and encouragement—vital concepts for living well.

Volunteering is certainly one way to serve others, but even before you decide to head over to the soup kitchen, take a look around your neighborhood or street or immediate group of acquaintances. I guarantee you there are people in your life you can connect with. But you have to generate enough momentum and risk just a little.

Do you know a young couple on your street with kids? You know they could use a break or a night out because they're in the mean years (i.e. kids under ten). I'm sure they would feel like they'd just won the lottery if you offered to babysit or pay for a sitter so they could take a night off and go to dinner without the kids in tow.

There are so many ways we can be thoughtful and mindful of other people. I don't care if it's helping somebody jump their car or carry their groceries. There are opportunities everywhere. Look for people who need help in little ways. It will start to change what you see in the world. If we don't look, we won't see the need.

When we're actively looking for ways to help others, we become less focused on what burdens we carry or what we have and don't have. We see a role open up that only we can fill, one that benefits others in their time of need and has that residual effect of making our own life that much brighter. That's the secret about serving others; sometimes we get more in return than we ever thought possible.

At our core, we are built to be with others. We were made to be in relationships. We need them. And yes, it's hard to do that in chapters that are difficult. But please, take a risk and trust me; it may be the first step in getting the life back that you feel is gone.

# WHAT DO YOU VALUE?

One of my main goals in writing this book is to help you find greater meaning in life while accepting and managing the challenges that come with it. Struggle well and live well.

Yes, life is a complicated beast, and even the best advice in the world isn't going to solve every problem we encounter. But if I could leave you with one piece of advice, something so fundamentally important to making the most of your time here on planet Earth, it would be this: live your life by your values. A value is something we intentionally act upon because it gives our life a sense of purpose and consistency.

Critical to living by our values is defining what those values are. We can ask ourselves questions like, "What kind of friend or family member do I want to be?" or "What life skills do I want to develop?" These will help us identify what's important to us and more clearly define our values.

Values are ongoing actions that we choose to perform or neglect at any given moment. No matter how happy or unhappy we are; no matter how in or out of love we are; and no matter how successful or unsuccessful we are at our job, we always have the choice to live by our values.

Values might include caring for a spouse, being a trustworthy colleague, maintaining a nutritious lifestyle, living a life that reflects our spirituality, giving time and money to those less fortunate, or even finding new ways to have fun. The most important thing is to figure out what we value and pursue it.

When we choose to act on our values, we take the first conscious steps down a brighter, clearer road where meaning, opportunity, and purpose await. That's what life is all about, and that's a life worth living.

# CHAPTER
## four

# SEASONS

# LIFE IS ABOUT CHANGE—BOTH GOOD AND BAD

The hard part about life is that it's constantly changing, whether we accept the change or not. One moment we're fist bumping the car salesman as we drive our new fully-loaded, 4-wheel drive beast off the lot; the next we're scraping the bottom of our piggy banks for lunch money and drunk dialing our ex-girlfriends or ex-boyfriends. And we think, "Man, I never thought I'd be here in life. I thought the good job and the happy family were permanent. I thought everything would stay the same."

Life isn't just a box of chocolates. Life is an inconsistently cyclical amalgamation of conditions engendered by uncontrollable combinations of inputs and outputs populated by an infinite number of boxes of chocolates. Whew! Not very sexy, is it? Well, here's an easier definition: life has seasons.

If you think of life in seasons, you'll start to understand a few important things. You'll realize that it's probably best to enjoy the good seasons while they last, because they don't. And we have to be active in our thoughts about the joys of the good seasons. If you start talking about the season ending before it's over, you're robbing yourself of the joy of the season. Don't. And when you're in the middle of those bad seasons, it's good to remember that those seasons don't last either; things do get better.

I have always loved biographies, reading or watching someone talk about their life unfolding. There is so much wisdom about life when we see it all unfold as one uninterrupted season. Right now I'm in Nelson Mandela's story—amazing man. And he would tell you with a smile and sweet accent that the chances your life will change are one hundred percent. I think he would tell you, and I would tell you, don't dread the "what now?" Embrace it like you expected it: you should—it will come. And know that you can do this and that the next chapter just might be the most epic and amazing one of your life. It was for Mandela.

Life is all about change. We can either succumb to that miserable feeling every human experiences when things change, or we can persevere, adapt, and take everything we can out of the current season. We're actually pretty good at dealing with reality when we make the effort.

If you're unhappy with the season you're in, don't just sit back and wait for it to change. Do something about it. You have that power. And when you learn to embrace the new chapter in your life, pretty soon that season of misery makes way for a season of joy.

Or maybe you're experiencing the best season of your life. Your kids are doing well in school, you and your spouse are communicating in more ways than one, you love your job, and the dog has stopped destroying your bedroom when you're away. Soak it up like it will never end. Enjoy every breath of it. Wake up early and stay up late. And yes, it won't always be like this. And that's okay. Your kids are going to leave one day, you and your spouse are going to fight, you might lose your job, and the dog could catch a whiff of the beef jerky you left next to your pillow. Seriously, who eats beef jerky before bedtime?

# ARE YOU KIDDING ME?

This entry is the result of countless discussions and observations. Like many things in this book, it has also been a joy to watch this in my own life and those close to me. It makes me laugh, and it makes me sigh and look at my lovely bride and ask, "How did we do it?" And yes, she always looks at me with the same puzzled expression and says, "I don't know." As husbands, wives, fathers, and mothers already know, the stages of married life can get particularly challenging. Let's walk through them together.

### The carefree years

In the early years of marriage, before children, couples experience an unparalleled time of devotion to each other and the ability to enjoy all that life has to offer married couples. It's a time to travel, experience foods and places, and begin relationships that last a lifetime.

We can decide to go to the 7:30 pm movie at 7:20 pm. We can say "yes" to the lake with friends on a Friday at 5:30 pm. Ah yes, freedom and a zest for living the abundant life.

### The mean years

Yes, I love my kids. I'm so glad to have them. How-damn-ever, it is a shock to the marital bliss when they invade. If you have children between the ages of newborn and ten years old, you've reached the "mean years." Why mean? Because these little bundles of joy have no ability to sustain life. Once they're able to feed themselves and rummage through pantries and drawers, we falsely hope that they'll have the ability to dress themselves and care for themselves. Yeah, wrong.

During this period you are prone to say to your kids something like, "Hey, run get dressed, we're going to see Mimi," only to look up and realize they're dressed like Batman or Tinker Bell or are wearing snow boots in July. While they're capable of grabbing clothes, they have no ability to grab appropriate clothes or even put them on the right way. They depend on you for their existence.

These are draining years for parents. It seems like you barely have enough energy to care for these little bundles of joy (and they are bundles of joy, but they drain your battery). Once they're fed, bathed, and down for the evening, there's little battery left to address your other adult responsibilities, like watching after the home, paying bills, and just trying to reintroduce yourself to that other bleary-eyed person across the table. Sex and time with each other become low priorities. And it's not uncommon in this season of life to hit a brick wall when it comes to nutrition, sleep, and exercise. These are brutal years on parents.

But, to be fair, they are also some of the most adorable years, probably some of the best pictures and most precious moments with your children. The innocence and joy is contagious. It is a wonderful time to watch and be with them. Soak it up. And hang in there; it gets better. Slowly.

### The busy years
These are the years from age ten to leaving for college/getting a job and moving out of the house. There is a sense of marginal success. They now have the ability to feed themselves. Even if they're not always eating the best food, it does bring relief that you no longer have to cut things into small pieces and you might even get to eat your own meal while it's still warm. It's the first glimmer of hope for a new future. Shortly thereafter, it dawns on you that they're old enough to practice sports and get involved in extracurricular activities. The problem? You are their transportation.

And in the midst of homework, practice, parties, and laundry, they are beginning to form the structure of their personality. They have the ability to express thoughts and feelings, honing the art of disagreement and sarcasm. Navigating the dangers of adolescent relationships, sex, substances, and homework is no easy work. They are also learning from experience as well as instruction. It can be demanding, emotional work for both parents and children.

You then find yourself shuttling rambunctious adolescents back and forth. It feels as if you live in your car. While not as draining as the mean years, it's an extraordinarily busy time. They're able to engage in conversations and step into challenges that give you hope for the future. It's a wonderful time, but make no mistake, you're busier than you've ever been in your life.

What's the first sign that there may be a life worth living after the busy years? One of your kids turns sixteen, and you have a designated driver. You have a little relief and hope for the future.

### The milk and honey years

If you're lucky, the kids will graduate high school, possibly college, and find employment. If you're fortunate, they will move out of your house. This is the time for you and your spouse to put more wood on the fire. Have an adventure together, do something new. This could be one of the most rewarding and meaningful chapters of your married life. Make no mistake, it takes energy, but it's worth it. At this point, we've learned to sacrifice more, think of ourselves less, and if we're lucky, have a better outlook on life.

And yes, there are plenty of challenges in these years. Health and retirement and career start to change, some coming to an end. Your parents' health may begin to fade, and you find yourself parenting parents. But somehow it's different; you are different. And if your marriage survives, it may be different in a way that amazes you.

So if you're a new parent, you've been warned: the mean years are coming. And they will be followed by the busy years. But take heart, the season of milk and honey is just around the bend. And it is sweet; oh, it is sweet.

# YOUR NEW YEAR'S RESOLUTION: BE HEALTHIER (PERIOD!)

I'm big on resolutions. I'm big on picking a date to start an event.

New Year's Day, unfortunately, is a day that a lot of people select. And it matches where they're at in the change process. They've been thinking about improving their health for months. But there are a *lot* of people who line up mid-December and go, "Yeah, me, too. I'll join the gym," with the guy who has been thinking about it for three, four, or five months.

But here's the catch: the "me, too" crowd on January 1 will be out of that gym by February. Go to any gym in January and you're going to see people you'll never see again. You'll see them wearing their brand new clothes, doing stuff on machines that they shouldn't be doing. And they'll be gone by February. Why? Because they were "me, too" people.

Here are a couple of tips on picking dates, because choosing the right date is important. First, setting a date in the future means you'll have time to be ready with head *and* feet. Second, before it arrives, make some little changes, adjustments in your routines, and know that you're going to commit to the date you picked and step into the effort on that day. Third, we know from experience that we'll meet the date if we share it with a few people. Not on the Internet, but in person. Share your plan and the date with a few people. Be accountable. Step out and try it. That mindset helps us achieve goals.

Finally, to keep our resolution manageable and achievable, we have to be able to measure what it is we're trying to do. Picking a date helps us get started. It also helps shift our mindset to, "I'm ready for this. I've thought about this a lot. I can do this." We're more likely to accomplish our goal because now we've got some skin in the game. Even when we falter, we're apt to say to ourselves, "That's okay; this is challenging, but I've got this. This is where I'm at, and I'm going to follow through."

If we're not able to follow through on our goal, then we need to step back. "Maybe I wasn't as ready to change this as I thought. Maybe there are some other things at play that I haven't considered." It doesn't mean we've abandoned our goal, but maybe our approach needs to change a little. So, if you pick a date in January to start and you're not really ready, don't do it.

Instead, examine the goal that you have set for yourself. Take a big-picture look. Understand that we do better when we have short-term goals and long-term goals that are objective and can be measured. We want a plan that anybody can look at and say, "Okay, I see how you are going to measure success." Just "feeling better" is something we can't measure. "Looking better" is something we can't measure, either.

But we know we've made progress when we can now wear the old suit we bought or fit into the new dress or our "skinny jeans." That's an achievable goal. It doesn't always have to be numbers, but numbers do help. The short-term goal may be that we're going to eat three fewer portions or drink three fewer cans of soda each week. For the month, it may be that we substitute half of the meals we usually eat takeout and instead make nutritious meals we've cooked at home. Maybe the monthly goal is to walk or run three more miles than last month.

If we've set a goal that we think and feel is hopeless, we should break it up into pieces. *(Remember that entry early on in this book, Break It Up.)* Don't look at the end goal and get overwhelmed. Just take that off the table. Our goal is to be better than we were yesterday. And if our goal is to be better than yesterday, we might just think we can do it. That little change can be the impetus to get started or to stay at it.

If what keeps you stuck is the thought that you have tried to change something and haven't been successful, or you are just afraid you can't do it, don't let those feelings keep you trapped. The fear of failure is not nearly as terrifying as the fear of never taking that step forward. If you are going to fear anything, fear not trying. Failure is just information you need to succeed the next time.

So, look at a goal for this week and maybe a goal for a month. Start on a goal for today and set a goal for the week. Start small and build on it because success is contagious.

# STOP HATING VALENTINE'S DAY

Ladies, here's a little secret about Valentine's Day.

When it's just us guys in the room and women are out of earshot, we take a vote. Nine out of ten of us agree that Valentine's Day is just a made-up holiday for us to do things for our wives and girlfriends because we didn't do enough for them on other holidays.

But what about that one-out-of-ten kind of guy who thinks Valentine's Day should be federal law?

Usually he's the fella who loves his wife so much that he'll sit through an entire season of *Grey's Anatomy* without complaining. He's the kind of guy who makes the rest of us look bad because the rest of us weren't willing to step away from Monday Night Football to answer a call from our wives.

We may roll our eyes at the poor sap, but—it may be time to take a page from that playbook and start recognizing the value in celebrating a day devoted to your significant other. And, yes ladies, please remember that this day is about celebrating your guy as well.

The problem is that we ourselves have perpetuated this idea that Valentine's Day is some goopy, flower-fueled, chocolate-covered lovefest. That's right, we're to blame.

It's not that women don't like flowers or chocolates, because plenty do. It's that we don't know how to do any better.

We haven't figured out that Valentine's Day isn't just about saying "I love you," which most of us say every single day anyway. Valentine's Day is about a very concrete thing. It's about showing gratitude. It's about saying thank you.

You know you're doing Valentine's Day right when you're doing something to say, "Thank you for being supportive in my life. Thank you for your companionship. Thank you for letting me share my life with you. Thank you for sharing your life with me."

It's also an opportunity to foster a tenderness that many marriages have lost. I see this with every couple that struggles, a loss of tenderness that we show to people in the office or at a restaurant but not to our spouses. Bringing that attitude home can go a long way to reconnecting.

One of the most common problems in long-term relationships is that we grow complacent. Seeing each other every day, taking trips together, eating together, and waking up together can be an exciting prospect for newlyweds, but for marriage veterans being together so much breeds complacency.

Valentine's Day is the perfect time to say thank you, to express gratitude for the role your partner plays in your life, and to say, "I'd pick you all over again."

# WHY JULY 4ᵀᴴ MATTERS EVERY DAY

Every summer we gather together, light the grill, eat too much, and set off fireworks all in the name of freedom and independence—concepts that are quintessentially American.

And, yes, let's admit it: there's a level of arrogance that comes from striking out on your own, in declaring that you don't need any helping hands except for the two at the ends of your arms. But with that also comes a frightening dose of vulnerability.

When the Founding Fathers let England know that they were moving out, I'm sure that they marched away with their heads held high and a quiver in their chins. They wanted freedom, and that's what they got: Freedom to triumph or freedom to fail. And don't you just know that King George & Co. watched them go with a curled lip and ill wishes? The little brother, thumbing his nose at his longtime protector, saying that he can do it better by himself.

Against all odds, America *did* do better all by itself. Today, it is one of the wealthiest and most powerful nations in the world, and it is also the one with the most freedom.

*Free.* It's a word that lives in everyone's mind: *I am* free *to say this; I am* free *to think that; I am* free *to be.* It has become such a part of who we are that it's practically woven into our skin the minute we're born. It's not so much American arrogance as American identity. We are also free to make this America better, and that's a freedom that seems to be shaky at the moment.

Take, for instance, a summer trip I once took to Italy. I was forty years old and not new to the world by any stretch of the imagination, and yet, I found myself turning to the friend I was visiting and saying, ''Oh, y'all don't really celebrate the Fourth of July over here, do you?''

And it's embarrassing to admit, because even though I had a rational thought nudging in the back of my head saying, *Of course they don't celebrate the Fourth of July!* I also had a much louder thought saying, *How could you not celebrate the day of America's Independence?*

We all carry America and all that it represents—home, freedom, triumph, and destiny—around with us wherever we go, tucked into our DNA.

There's a strength there that radiates from us, even some two hundred plus years after our Declaration of Independence was first written, that speaks to insurmountable odds that can be conquered.

# LISTEN FOR THE SPIRIT OF CHRISTMAS—ALL YEAR LONG

**S**anta is dead.

Okay, glad that's out of the way.

Actually, this comes from a discussion we had around the office one day this summer. "How do I deal with Santa Claus and my spirituality?" I know, strange having a discussion about Santa in the Texas heat, but when you have kids, that kind of thing happens.

Let's face it, there are some of us who can't hold the Baby Jesus and sit on Santa's lap at the same time. This conflict of religion and secularism (or commercialism) is a very real crisis for many of us, especially young parents. Just ask any elementary school teacher.

I just so happen to know an elementary school teacher really well, and this is a true tale from her class-room. One set of parents, a bit rigid in their thinking, told their son "Billy" that "there's no such thing as Santa." Of course Billy, in an effort to cling to the idea of a magical man who brings presents every year, responded, "Well, Cindy's parents told her there is a Santa!"—to which Billy's parents replied, "Well, Cindy's parents are lying to her." Life is so entertaining; you can't make this stuff up.

It didn't take any time for Billy to spread the story about Santa's demise around the classroom. And just like that, Santa was dead for a classroom of former believers. A small part of their childhood seemed lost forever.

All of this came full circle for me recently when I was watching *The Polar Express*. Remember in the movie how the parents can't hear Santa's sleigh bell? Only the kids can hear the bell. At the risk of overdoing the psychology of it all, it's symbolic of not being able to hear the Spirit of Christmas. Of not believing anymore.

What does this mean for us? Somewhere along the way of growing up, some of us have forgotten how to play, how to have fun, how to "believe" in something magical. We've lost the connection with our childhood. So my question during the holiday season is, "When did we lose that ability to play?"

At Christmastime, it's important to keep things in perspective. Santa only visits once a year. The whole event is an exciting time for children that tends to fade as soon as all of the gifts are opened and the decorations are stored away. Religion, on the other hand, can change lives and instill joy every day of the year. It's important to remember that Santa and religion don't have to be mutually exclusive, even if just one of them has a real shot at sustaining us after the presents have been opened.

The next time you hear a group of kids talking about Santa Claus, listen to what they have to say. Take note of their excitement and their pure joy during this magical time of year. Maybe, just maybe, it'll rekindle the fun of the season you once loved.

And, most certainly, feel free to also celebrate the more meaningful reason for the season—which, if you're open to it, can last all year long. I think you might just be able to do both.

# ALL THINGS IN MODERATION, INCLUDING MODERATION

When did moderation become a four-letter word?

We struggle with moderation. There seems to be an intrinsic desire in us to consume as much as absolutely possible. This appetite seems to have grown recently, fed by our instantly gratified lifestyles. And it's a long list of things we struggle with—food, tobacco, alcohol, drugs, sex, exercise, work, social media, and spending. Those are just some of the popular ones.

Think about it; we can order almost anything we want online and have it delivered to us the next day—or sooner! Consumer culture tells us that it's ludicrous that we should ever have to wait for anything, and we should never go home from a store empty-handed.

I was on vacation and saw a pair of shoes I wanted, but the store didn't have my size. When I got back to the hotel, I went on Amazon, found my size, and had the shoes delivered to my hotel two days later. That's insane! Half the reason I did it was sheer fascination with the process.

One of the main causes of our excess comes when we ask *things* to do something for us. That typically involves moving past moderation and taking the first step down the path of excess.

When we ask food to make us feel more relaxed, when we ask alcohol to make us feel less anxious, or when we ask shopping to make us feel good, then we're crossing into a dangerous place. When I talk with people who find themselves struggling with excessive use of things, there is almost always a problem in another area of their life that is not being addressed. They have a life problem, not an alcohol or food problem.

Too often we think of moderation as deprivation, when in reality it's a very healthy place to be. But when we have moved to a place of being excessive, course-correcting to a more appropriate consumption feels very different, uncomfortable even. If we are wrestling with moderation, it may be telling us something very important. Telling us that we are asking this external thing—be it food, alcohol, drugs, sex, spending—to do something for us, help us forget something, or distract us from the chaos in our lives.

But there are absolutely times when being excessive is perfectly appropriate and necessary if it's directed to a positive, goal-oriented effort. Achieving great things takes intensity! If you want to run a marathon, get a promotion, or score a second date with that special someone, moderation won't serve you very well. As long as you're practicing healthy behavior and working towards a healthy goal, being excessive can be the right approach. Because sometimes even moderation should be practiced in moderation.

There are moments in life for moderation and moments for going for it in a big way. Knowing the exact reasons why you're buying/drinking/saying/doing will help you determine whether you should practice moderation or go all out. If you find yourself in excess, slow down long enough to get a handle on your emotions, thoughts, and life. If your "escape" is getting out of hand, it may be time to rein it in. It's times like these that you need a few close people to help you see the situation better, because they usually can.

# CHAPTER five

# WORK

# NEVER RETIRE

I'm all about work. Not the communistic, do-it-for-the-greater-good-and-starve-while-doing-it kind of work. I'm an advocate of solid, meaningful work, the kind that connects you to people, stirs your passion for the job, and keeps you healthy.

I know all kinds of people who have been financially successful in business and have retired at a very young age. Of that group of retirees, the ones I see struggling the most with depression and addiction are the ones who don't stay engaged in meaningful work.

That drop from ultra-productivity to zero productivity can be a real kick in the gut.

On the other hand, I've interacted with millionaires and billionaires, people who literally don't need to work another day in their lives, who keep punching in every morning. I am fascinated by them and how their approach to work and life serves them to the end of their days.

It turns out that even when meaningful work is no longer a financial necessity, it remains an emotional, intellectual, and physical necessity.

The self-made men and women of the world still work because deep down they still need to, and that's not a bad thing. Some of them are older—in their seventies and eighties—and many of them have more energy and vitality than a lot of forty- and fifty-year-olds I know. These people understand that work doesn't have to be a dreaded obligation. Work can be something you pursue passionately that gives you energy on a daily basis.

To be clear, the message here is consistent, meaningful work, not overworking.

The key is to find meaningful work that's not going to break your back but will keep you engaged in your field of expertise or in the subject you feel most passionate about. Regardless of what you are doing, make sure it is something that is a talent, a gift. Something that you enjoy and could do all day and even forget to eat at times because you are so engaged. It's those things that give us energy and fill us with life. So, pursue those activities throughout the course of your life.

There's nothing like coming home with a sense of making a contribution, of being needed, or filling a role, however small or great. That satisfaction can be the best night of sleep you've ever had. Stop thinking about retirement and think about your next job—not a new career, just a job (or activity) that keeps you young.

# EVERY GREAT ACHIEVEMENT REQUIRES SACRIFICE

It doesn't matter how we measure achievement. For some, it's finishing high school. For others, it's completing college or graduate school. For some, it's having children and raising them (yes, you have to do both). For others, it's a career. It may be a physical challenge like a marathon or an IRONMAN®. For others, it may be finishing a yoga class (yep, this one's mine).

But if we're going to dare to do something great, we're going to have to make sacrifices, and some of our strivings will require greater sacrifices than others.

When we sacrifice to achieve, we learn and grow as people. If our goals don't lie just outside our reach, then we're never really going to have a chance to struggle and grow. No matter what type of goal we set, we're going to have to step away from things that make us comfortable, which gives us a chance to prioritize and to practice mental strength and discipline. Nothing wrong with comfortable, it's a great place to be at certain times and stages of life. However, we can grow complacent and stagnant if we're not careful.

Delaying our impulsivity and our desire for immediate gratification (two character attributes of many Americans) is a positive thing. And sometimes that means less time with our kids or spouse. It may mean we do a great job at work, not a perfect one.

Some of the things we strive for will cost us some of our comforts, like a peaceful existence or a sense of serenity. It's good for us to challenge ourselves at times.

To be candid, it's one of the reasons I do some of the ridiculous physical things that I do. I've learned that when we challenge ourselves physically, we're also challenging ourselves mentally. And it's in that space that we begin to see where our strengths and vulnerabilities are, where our growth points are.

## If we don't challenge ourselves, we won't grow.

Something to keep in mind: when you're in the midst of attempting to do something great, don't complain. If you've set off on a course to do something great, you should expect to suffer. It's a normal part of the process. Don't fight it, don't resist it, and don't be surprised by it; just roll with it. It's normal; it's appropriate. It's also probably temporary.

# THE FALSE ADVERTISING OF ANXIETY

If you were ever to make a case for false advertising, anxiety is the place to start. I don't know of a place where thoughts and feelings disappoint more than anxiety. And left unchecked, anxiety can wreak havoc on our work performance, relationships, and all-around peace of mind.

We can trace the anxiety in our lives to three main sources. The first is the "grain of truth"—not uppercase Truth, just lowercase, pea-sized truth. An example of a grain of truth is that story your Uncle Ralph posted on Facebook about the time he got bit by a rattlesnake.

Now, even though he shouldn't have been walking in a Texas field during summer in the first plan and even though the chances someone would actually get tagged by a rattlesnake is one in a million, the fact of the matter is that the snake *did* bite him. Next thing you know, social media has exploded with articles about how to guard against the all too common rattlesnake bite. Yes, I think social media has magnified this issue significantly. We used to only hear about things in our immediate circle of family and community. Now, we hear and see video from halfway around the world.

Instead of keeping the perspective that there's a one-in-a-million chance of getting bitten, our brains turn it into "there's a good chance it could happen." And that's what anxiety does; it distorts reality. It makes being out in nature a tense and fearful experience. It can steal joy in a heartbeat. Trust me, it does.

The second source of anxiety is our past. If our thoughts move to things that have either happened to us, our family, our friends, or people we know of, then we pull those past experiences into the present and act as if they are going to happen again.

Before we know it, we start behaving as if our thoughts and feelings are the truth. Our thoughts and feelings are true, but they are not the truth.

The third source of anxiety is the future. Many times anxiety brings a future possibility into the present and disguises it as a certainty. We feel and think and act as if we don't need to wait for life to happen, we know how it will play out. And it's never good. Which seems really biased, in a negative direction.

I've talked to many people who were in constant fear of losing their job because of some future mistake they might make. My first question is always very basic: "Why are you worried about losing your job?"

They might say, "A buddy of mine at work got fired. I can't believe he lasted this long, honestly. But they told him he had two weeks to finish up. How is he going to make house payments and car payments? Just like that he has no income. I can't do that. I have a wife and kids, and my wife would lose her mind if I lost my job. We would be homeless, literally." So I'll ask, "How will you become homeless?" And they'll answer, "If I don't have a job, I can't pay my bills; then I can't make mortgage payments, and then I'll be on the street."

Possibilities begin flooding out of them. They must have really good reasons to fear losing their jobs, right?

And yet, when I ask them about their employment history, it turns out that they've never been fired from a job, they've been working for the same company for seven years, they've become an integral part of the team, their coworkers find them fair and easy to work with, and they play Words with Friends® with the boss during breaks.

Isn't it funny how we sometimes get the impression that bankruptcy, homelessness, misfortune, and tragedy are lurking at our doorstep because of a single unsubstantiated thought?

Anxiety feeds off of passive thinking. When we think passively, we allow horrible, catastrophic thoughts to run around in our heads unchecked as if, number one, they're true, and, number two, they're having no impact on us.

To get out of this mess, we must be more active in our evaluation of our thoughts. We have to identify the source of our anxiety and then evaluate and challenge the thoughts that go through our heads to determine just how truthful those thoughts really are. Chances are the thoughts are not truthful at all.

Only then will we have the best chance of reducing our anxiety and opening our eyes to options and outcomes we didn't see before. We need our best thinking, and a head full of fears and "what ifs" is not going to provide our best thinking.

# FAILURE TO LAUNCH

At twenty-two years of age and sporting a college degree, your son or daughter decides that home is officially the best place to be, so they move back in.

What joy! Some of us have only dreamed of being able to spend so much time with our kids. Truly, this must be a gift from the heavens.

Curb your enthusiasm because the next thing you know they'll be twenty-nine years old with a beer gut living it up in the guest house.

Or worse, they'll decide to sit on the couch all day devouring cheese balls while combing through stacks of the VHS tapes you used to record *Full House* in 1990. Yeah, you've got a failure to launch problem.

You say to yourself, "Well, if they could just find a job."

This may come as a surprise, but they've already got a job, probably the best job in the world. Between food money, clothes money, gas money, and party money, they get paid the equivalent of, let's say, $40,000 a year for doing absolutely nothing. That's a whole lotta money for a whole lotta nothing. Where do I sign up?

If you don't want me moving into your house, you're probably going to have to give me some tough love, just like you're going to have to do with your own adult. (You expected to see me write kid, I know; they still feel like kids. They're not. They're full-grown adults.). And the only way to do that is to get on the same page with your spouse about what the expectations for your children should be.

It's likely that little Cindy or little Gary is exploiting the differences between you and your spouse in order to stay at home and veg out. Both of you may want your kid out of the house, but only one of you is feeding the habit. All your kid has to do is use an emotional—and patently illogical—argument that will make the parent with the weakest constitution bend like a Twizzler®. If they can fool at least one parent, chances are they've scored a permanent stay at Hotel Mom & Dad.

To combat this, parents have to get on the same page. I often tell parents, "Look, I don't care how pissed you are at each other; when you talk to your kid, I want you to sit on the couch as close to each other as possible. I want you to hold hands. I want you to create this physical, impassable wall. I guarantee your kid is not going to hear a word you say because he's going to be so freaked out that his parents are actually on the same page for once."

If you're still having trouble with the idea of pushing your kid out into the real world, just know that one of the least loving things you can do as a parent is feed a habit. If you truly want your kid to thrive, you have to get them out into the world and give them a chance to make it on their own. That's how you set them up for long-term success.

We're not like plants; we have to move to grow. Getting out of the house and doing something that requires effort, and even a little action, is what engages us with the world and with other people. It keeps us from becoming isolated and gives us hope, encouragement, and the belief that your life and my life could dramatically improve if we put a little effort into it.

Even if we have to give up the best job in the world to do it.

# PRINCIPLES OVER PEOPLE

Imagine you've got two daughters. You instruct daughter one to take out the trash. A week later, the trash still hasn't been taken out. You're furious, but then you remember that daughter one likes making you breakfast in bed on Saturday mornings. How could you punish someone who cooks the perfect omelet? So, you let it slide.

The next week you instruct daughter two to take out the trash. A week later, the trash still hasn't been taken out, and you start wondering what kind of Kool-Aid® of Disobedience your daughters have been drinking.

You march upstairs to daughter two's bedroom and ground her on the spot. You have no trouble grounding daughter two because she never makes you breakfast in bed. She's also got this weird thing she does with her nose . . . anyway, grounding her was the right thing to do.

No, go ahead, pat yourself on the back because you just scarred one of your children for life by picking favorites.

That's what happens when we choose people over principles. You laid out your expectations for both daughters, but only one of your daughters felt the consequences for disobeying. Now, daughter two doesn't understand why you love daughter one more, and worse, you get the sinking feeling that one day daughter two will no longer return your phone calls and "have plans" for Christmas and not make it this year.

The same goes for the workplace, especially if you're in a management position.

Maybe you've got an assistant manager that's constantly making inappropriate or borderline comments about everything from women to race to politics, but you don't really say anything to him because he's one of your top performers. Later, you find out another assistant manager is saying the same kinds of things, only this guy doesn't bring in as much revenue as your golden boy. If you fire this guy and your employees find out you didn't fire the other guy, you're going to find yourself in deep water. You start to lose credibility, and people start to question how decisions are made.

People don't trust leaders who are unfair. People don't function optimally when they're not sure who their boss is going to punish or not punish and for what reasons.

Honesty and integrity are principles by which we should live and die. When we put principles before people, we gain others' trust and avoid the fallout of poor decision-making.

Simply put, people prefer to follow leaders who are consistent in what they say and how they act. They follow leaders who are not afraid to do the right thing, regardless of who the person is. No, it's not some kind of idealized standard. Look at great leaders and look at great people; it's one of the things that make them great.

Principles give us a kind of compass that helps us excel in a complex and demanding world. When we live by principles, we save ourselves a lot of heartache and confusion; decisions generally get easier to make; and the standard to which we hold ourselves accountable becomes clearer.

So, stick to your guns. Fire both managers if their actions justify it. Ground both of your daughters when they fail to follow through on what was agreed. I don't care if your daughter is the next Emeril Lagasse; always maintain your principles. Even if there's bacon involved.

# WORK-LIFE BALANCE: CREATE YOUR NEW NORMAL

The good old days when a company only had to offer job candidates a nice insurance and 401k package are gone. Workers today (thanks in part to the injection of Millennials into the work-force) are looking for additional perks like extended time off, tuition reimbursement, even on-site childcare centers.

Their objective? To find a balance between their work and personal life.

But is work-life balance a real thing or just some dream with unicorns and rainbows? Just ask yourself these questions: Do you find yourself feeling fatigued before, during, and after work? Do your thoughts drift in and out of work-related matters even when you're at home? If you answered yes, your work may be spreading into your personal life like a bad weed. And that may end up in a case of work-life *imbalance*.

Now, to clarify, I'm not talking about the times when we have to suck it up and work long, hard hours for a season. Most jobs have that, some more than others—welcome to life. I'm not talking about those times; I'm talking about getting to a place where work is the vast majority and personal life is minimal.

And you're not alone! I guarantee some of your colleagues are probably dealing with the same thing. In the world of capitalism and connectivity, conditions like this are increasingly common.

It's not that capitalism has it in for us. The issue is our unwillingness to call it quits when the workday is over. I don't think there has ever been a time in "Corporate America" when this has been such a widespread issue. We have computers in our pockets that keep us tethered to our desk. They're even waterproof so we can take them to the beach when we're on vacation.

And yet, working more never really yields the results we want. More often than not, being a disciple of work means a decreased devotion to relationships, rest, and activities we love. And this level of neglect can be detrimental to our health and wellbeing.

There are, however, measures we can take to correct the imbalance, even when our workload seems endless.

First, we have to disengage. Maybe that means setting an electronic curfew. Or perhaps when we leave the office, we shut down our email. Because, if we really want to put our lives back into balance, we have to make a clear distinction between our work life and our personal life. Disengaging is the most effective approach.

Next, make a commitment to do something outside of work. It could be coaching a soccer team, walking the dog, taking an art class, or getting friends together for game night. Having a calendar marked up with enjoyable activities takes us out of the daily grind and gives us something to look forward to.

When we participate in those activities, it's important to be just as mentally present as we are physically present. Even when we're doing enjoyable things with people we love, our thoughts can easily drift back to all of those unanswered emails.

The remedy is to be wholly present with the people around you. Enjoy the activity to the fullest. Don't let your career and the stress it brings be a distraction from the time you've set aside to relax and recharge.

Maintaining work-life balance is all about keeping our personal lives separate from our business lives. We must learn to be more active in this area, intentionally letting calls go to voicemail, leaving email responses for the morning, and making our personal time a priority. Don't talk about about work-life balance, just quietly and effectively do it.

# CHAPTER
## SIX

# PLAY

# WHAT'S ON YOUR "PLAYLIST?"

I've learned that I have to protect play. I have to protect those times where I intentionally step away from the demands and chores of life because I know that play is critical to my health. And play is critical to *your* health as well. Just because most of us quit playing over time, this reality doesn't mean that we don't need it.

Play gives us balance in a society that demands we do our jobs with extreme effort and constant attention. Whether you work on the construction site or on the fiftieth floor of the Empire State Building, it can be so easy—tempting, even—to allow job-related stress and responsibilities to take over your life. That's where play comes in.

For you rebellious types, think of play as a way to fight the system. If we're going to fight the system, we have to be smart about it. Too much play is like having Christmas every day. After a week of opening presents and drinking your child's weight in eggnog, you'll find that the day starts to lose its specialness.

So, balance and moderation are key, once again. The other crucial thing we have to understand is what play really is. What counts as play and what doesn't?

First, take a look at your list—your "playlist," if you will. If wine and TV are the only two things on your playlist, then you may have a problem. The good news is that it's a solvable problem because chances are you like to do other things, too.

Maybe you enjoy reading fiction. Ignore the people who look down on fiction simply because they are too busy reading the latest management or career advice book and dust off your limited edition copy of *The Lord of the Rings*. Fiction is a place to get lost and engage with deep stories and characters who reflect our own human desires and shortcomings. And adventure, humans need adventure.

Second, don't fight the personal challenges that may surprise you as you step into play. It should happen, but learn from it. For instance, do you struggle with turning play into a job? Are you so competitive that you have lost any sense of enjoyment? And worse, are you out of touch with what you are doing in an activity in the midst of play? If you started bowling for fun and fellowship but ended up being the league chairman and spend countless hours organizing and scheduling, you may have turned play into a job.

In a world that constantly presents unique challenges and demands, play gives us a place to practice without paying a big price. It's an activity where we can take risks, manage the thoughts we have about the uncertainty of the task, and experience some failure and some success. Play was where we learned as kids to solve problems, create games that we still talk about, and try things that we would never have tried in life if we hadn't gotten some experience on the playground or in the fields near our house.

If you're really stumped about this whole "play" business, ask your kid or grandkid. Kids are really good at playing, and they'll probably even let you join.

And remember, time to play won't just show up on our calendar, anymore than spending time with the family will. You have to make time for play; and to make the most out of that time, you better get rid of any and all distractions, especially phones. Because perusing Facebook does *not* count as play.

# DON'T DO THAT

I'm not sure what to do, either.

I can't tell you how many times I think that or say that. And I work with some pretty incredible colleagues, some really bright men and women who know how to help people who are struggling. But there are times when we, the professionals, aren't even sure what the best course of action is.

One of the things I've realized in working with people is that there are a couple of ways to begin to break down a difficult situation. One that continues to serve me well is this: *I'm not sure what we should do, but I can dang sure tell you what we shouldn't do.* Knowing what not to do can be just as important as knowing what to do.

We've all been in that situation. We may be puzzled by what to do; but if it doesn't take much for us to start listing the things we know beyond a shadow of a doubt we should not do, then that's where we need to start. Make that list and title it "Don't Do This." As the "Don't Do This" list grows, the "Do This" list should be a little easier to identify.

When we get hung up on not knowing what to do, we can feel like nothing is being done or that we are lost in the process. It feels too big and insurmountable. Starting the list of Don't Do has an odd effect in helping us to feel we are making progress, like we have started to sort out this thing that has occupied our every waking moment. It breathes a little confidence in us that we can do this: we can start to put a strategy in place that will change our direction for the better.

You'll begin to notice that many times our emotions fill out the list of what we should do, while rational thinking will populate what we should not do. It's what people mean when they say, "You're doing it for all the wrong reasons," which is their way of saying this is a decision based on emotions—anxiety, sadness, lust, or loneliness. And that's our challenge. How do we blend logic and emotion when it comes to making important decisions in our lives? We can do it, and it starts with asking ourselves the question, "What should I *not* do?"

# YOU'RE BETTER WHEN YOU MOVE

The Greek philosopher Plato wrote, "In order for man to succeed in life, God provided him with two means—education and physical activity. Not separately, one for the soul and the other for the body, but for the two together. With these two means, man can attain perfection."

Yahtzee® for Plato! (For those game novices, this equates to rolling a perfect combination.)

If I could encourage you to do one thing to improve your life today, it would be to engage in some sort of physical activity.

Let me speak bluntly—and scientifically: We need to produce neurotransmitters. You heard me right.

Serotonin, norepinephrine, dopamine, and endorphins are naturally-occurring neurotransmitters in our bodies. And part of their purpose is to make us feel good! Like euphoria good. Yeah, they may sound like the names of tiny dwarves, but they play a giant role in making our boat float, putting the pedal to the metal, and igniting our afterburners. The production of these naturally-occurring stimulants is at its peak when we engage in physical activity, pleasurable activities. No, texting doesn't count. You have to get your heart rate up.

Physical activity changes our daily routine, increases our interactions with others, and helps us overcome physical and psychological challenges. When we keep after it, we begin to eat more carefully, which can lead to shedding that winter weight.

Let me repeat that. If you want to improve your mental health, get off your sedentary arse and get moving. Physical activity will give you a running head start to reduce your anxiety and negative mood and improve your self-esteem and cognitive function. Just move. It doesn't have to be at a gym, try a Zumba® class, or hot yoga or Pilates® session (all great stuff for some people). You can even just walk on your street or at the mall. A vigorous walk, not a shopping pace.

This is especially true if you struggle with depression, anxiety, or addiction. Drugs and alcohol leech our body of key nutrients and, over long periods, deteriorate the systems in our bodies. It's sort of like strip mining, which by the way, we have outlawed because it's bad for the earth. It's just as bad for the body.

Okay, okay, you say, "I don't need a lecture on exercise."

I'm not trying to guilt trip you, but I am sounding the alarm. When we need to heal our body, mind, and spirit, that healing comes sooner when we engage in meaningful physical activity. Now, don't ask physical activity to do more than it can. It is not an approved remedy for the treatment of cancer or high cholesterol. But we should expect exercise to do what it can and does: it plays a role in our happiness.

Start out small. Walk two blocks. Eat an apple or a banana for a snack. Drink three glasses of water during the day, more if you can. The little things add up! As you feel better, expand the intensity, frequency, and duration—walk longer, eat healthier more often, and drink that water up. Even one hour a week of physical activity will benefit your wellbeing!

And after a few weeks or months, you may even choose to begin exercising—physical activity that is planned, structured, repetitive, and performed with the goal of improving health or fitness on a sustained basis.

Just call me Plato.

Okay, don't.

# ACCEPTING THE WONDERFUL WORLD OF IMPERFECT

Nobody. Not one person. Not your hero, not your sainted aunt, not your parents. Not your teacher, preacher, or trainer, either.

No one is perfect.

No one is going to perfectly get, create, or fulfill all of our wants and needs. Now, most will read that and agree and feel like I am a profound observer of the obvious. However, that is not how the perfection bug works. It's like advertising. I love it when people watch a commercial and say, "I don't get it, that doesn't work on me." Yeah, it does.

Now, let me unpack perfectionism a bit.

Perfectionism can ruin our lives. Not only does our quest for perfectionism contribute significantly to high levels of stress and pressure, but it also leads to anxiety, lower self-esteem, lower confidence, and an overall lower quality of life. And when we expect others to be perfect, we're just setting ourselves up for heartbreak. At its extreme, perfectionism can lead to burnout and breakdowns.

So what's the cure to living with Perfection Infection?

#1: Define Terms. Perfection is an *opinion*. We change our minds all the time. So, we have to change our minds about what we have to do to be "perfect" in our lives, which we already established we can't be. Instead of "perfect," consider using the word "well."

Example: "I would like to do that well." This is the kind of well as in, "Shake well before using."

#2: Play. Done well, playing is the antidote to perfectionism. Playing is about creating a space in our lives where we really don't have to accomplish anything. Where there is no need to accomplish, there is virtually no need to strive for perfection. Every workday is already geared toward accomplishing something, whereas playing a game for recreation is geared toward having fun. Remember *fun?* It alleviates stress and pulls us out of our daily mission to win at all costs.

#3: Listen to your imperfections. Our imperfections can serve a purpose if we accept them. People relate and connect to others more easily when they don't feel like they must be perfect. We know the opposite is true: "Perfect people" have few friends.

When we're okay with our imperfections, we'll relax, smile, and enjoy work and life more. That sounds like a perfectly imperfect life!

# GIVE ME A BREAK

If you were able to survive high school or college without the use of a cell phone or computer, you will completely understand this one. If you're under thirty, you've already turned the page.

True story. The other day I had to make a quick run to the grocery store. I backed out of my driveway and realized I didn't have my phone. I stopped in the street, frozen like a Popsicle® trying to think about what to do. I had a lengthy conversation in my head about the dangers of leaving without my phone. Then it hit me, "This is ridiculous. I've lived most of my life without a cell phone." So I sped off to the store without it (yes, I drive too fast sometimes).

It amazes me how easily our pocket computers (a.k.a. cell phones) have stolen our quiet times.

New apps and gadgets are supposed to make our lives easier, or at least they're marketed that way. But we all know that technology has made our lives more hectic and fast-paced. Whether it's a constant stream of emails that need answering or daily alerts about the latest Kanye "kantroversy," the information overload never seems to quit.

The solution, which isn't always easy, is to put a stop to it yourself. When it's playtime, put the phone away. Turn it off, silence it, lock it in a safe, do whatever you have to do to make sure nothing interrupts the precious time you've set aside for yourself and for your family.

Even if it's Mom calling, stay strong. Resist. You can call her back later if she doesn't call you again, which she will.

Our time away from work—and sometimes family—in whatever form it takes for an individual, is critical to our health. When we work, work, work, we stretch, stretch, stretch our bodies to limits where they weren't meant to function. So, is it really the job that's so terrible, or could it be that you lack the discipline to let things go to voicemail? Do you have trouble letting email sit until the morning? Are you the guy texting on "date night" because a colleague asked a question? I would hate for you to quit a job only to find out *you* are the problem, not the job.

Trust me, we have endless abilities to ruin every job we have.

So, stop complaining. Do you have any standards you set for yourself? Well, that's the first place to start. Actually, ask your spouse or kids if they think you are on your phone too much. Be careful, I asked my son the same question one day when he was about twelve. He was really sweet and intended no ill will when he said, "Yeah, people call you a lot." Right there, that moment, man it hurt. I'll never forget that. I committed to never answering my phone when I'm with my kids. If it's a true emergency, I tell them and ask if it's okay. But that almost never happens. We need commitments and standards or else we won't make progress.

Now, finish your list. What else are you going to have as a standard? No phones at meals? No texting in bed? Get to work; the life we want doesn't just happen. We have to plan it and develop it. And yes, we will struggle to get it right, but if we stay after it, we will live well.

Now excuse me while I go call my mom. I'm feeling the need to apologize for something.

# CHAPTER
## seven

# HELL

# ALCOHOL

**S**ure, have a beer.

Alcohol is not our problem. Neither is pot or pain medications. It doesn't matter how much or how little is available. It doesn't matter if it's legal or illegal. None of those things really bother me. Because, at the end of the day, *the problem is with people.*

Now I'm not saying I think we ought to legalize everything. As we've learned over the decades, sometimes government has to step in because, as a group, we can be really stupid. So yes, I think we need some restraints on what's available.

But think about it. Every outcome begins with choice.

I've spent quite a bit of my career with some tremendous researchers as well as treatment professionals who specialize in the area of addictions. I've learned that whether it's the first drink, the first cigarette, or the first pill, it always begins with a fairly harmless choice.

STRUGGLE WELL, LIVE WELL

And might I point out that the first time we taste alcohol, it tastes horrendous. Across the board, it's a bad taste. The first cigarette burns the hair out of your nose. And the first time you put a pinch of ground up tobacco in your mouth, well, let the spinning world commence!

Simple question: why do we keep doing it? Simple answer: it does something to us and for us.

When we start drinking alcohol for casual and social reasons, we can slowly but surely acquire a taste for it. Whether it's a beer with barbeque or wine with fish, we can acquire a taste and enjoy the taste. And by the way, the vast majority of people who do that will do so without any problems. I'm talking seventy to eighty percent of the people.

For reasons we don't fully understand some people continue in a compulsive way to schedule their day in order to drink. It seems to grow, it seems to get worse, and most of the time it doesn't get better without some serious effort put forth by the individual or from outside people.

It's because most of the time we're asking alcohol to do something for us. We get home from work and take a drink to forget about it. We start drinking in the afternoons because we're worn out from the kids and anticipate our husbands getting home. We get anxious before we meet with people, so we'll have one or two drinks to "take the edge off." If we do that enough, we will begin to think "I can't do that without having a drink." Talk about bad news beers.

The good news? People quit all the time. Yes, it's possible to get back the life you thought was lost because of alcohol or drug use. It's also true that you're going to have to mend some fences and rebuild some bridges. Unfortunately, there are some fences you can't mend, some bridges you can't rebuild. When you use substances in a way that starts to look like an addiction, you sometimes have to lie, mislead people, or even steal. One of the hardest things for people after they quit is realizing they no longer have to do those things. It can take years to overcome these behaviors.

Yeah, we humans struggle with things that alter our minds and moods. And we really struggle when substances lie to us and make us believe that we're relaxing and getting away from the stress of life. If we are honest, a drink or two does make us relax, take the edge off, and can help us forget about all that's going on with the kids. It works in the short run. Our problem is that we don't get the dose correct; we're usually increasing it to get the same effect.

If we start to use alcohol in greater amounts and more regularly than we used to and if we start to rely on it to calm our anxiety or help us forget our troubles, then we are down a path that starts to look like an addiction. A life that is out of control. But as strange as it sounds, our real problem is not with the alcohol. Most of the time we have a life problem that we are trying to solve with alcohol. Our problem is inside us.

And, it takes a conscious decision and day-by-day approach to resolve this life problem. It's time to develop the skills and change your thoughts and actions. Reading this book is a good first step and then implement these ideas to bring your life back into control. Now, if you find these changes too hard to tackle alone, maybe it's time to seek a bit more help from friends, a support group, or a therapist.

# THE CAKE DIDN'T EAT ITSELF

I love pizza.

If you've spent any time around me, it won't come as a surprise that I have the taste buds of a five-year-old. For some reason, I don't eat most vegetables, and I just don't care for a lot of foods. And, when it comes to a new food, please don't ask me to try it; I'm almost certain I have. I just don't like it. It's both a texture and a taste thing.

But over the past decade, having worked with organizations like the Cooper Clinic in Dallas, I've made it a point to eat healthier foods. (Side note, Dr. Cooper coined the term "aerobics," how cool is that?) After talking to nutrition experts, here's what I learned.

If the first rule of Fight Club is don't talk about Fight Club, then the first rule about being on a diet is don't talk about being on a diet. A diet is a list of what you can and can't do. It's just a bad way to set your mind up towards food. Talk about eating healthy. That's all you're really doing. Eating healthy is a life-long journey, whereas a diet is something we do for a week or a month or three months before returning to the promised lard—I mean *land*.

Over the past twenty-five years, we have seen an epidemic spreading across this country like no other. Obesity rates are sky-rocketing among adults and now children. What people don't seem to be drawing a connection to is that our increasing rates of joint pain, heart problems, diabetes, and cancers are very much related to obesity.

Much like problems with alcohol, obesity starts with a choice. No matter how you spin it, the cake (or in my case, the pizza) didn't eat itself.

To be fair, the food industry is not helping us out. First, the portion size on the plate in front of you is for a grizzly bear, not an average human. So the next time you're at dinner or at lunch, order a smaller portion, split with a friend, or take half of the meal to go. Learn what a portion size is; you'll be amazed at how it helps.

Slow down. We eat too fast and have bad habits around food. Prepare a meal on a plate rather than grazing around the kitchen. Sit down at a table and enjoy your food there instead of on the sofa by the television. Try to actually taste your food.

Stop believing things on labels. Prepackaged food is, by and large, not healthy food. If you're wondering what healthy food is, do a simple test. Go to the grocery store and buy food you think is healthy, bring it home, and see how long it takes for the food to go bad. If it doesn't go bad within the next three or four days, it's not healthy food. Healthy food is supposed to go bad. If it can sit on your shelf for two weeks and retain its youthful glow, fuhgetaboutit.

Lastly, monitor your intake of food and your burn rate of calories. It's just like keeping track of your income and expenses. Do the same with your calorie intake and how many calories you're burning. I promise you'll be more mindful of just how many calories are in that double macchiato. And don't fly off the rails trying to get into an elite gym or sport the newest fitness apparel. You don't have to join a CrossFit® class or trendy studio just to be physically active.

It all starts with a choice. Food has emotion tied to it. We find it soothing, comforting, and distracting. We have to be careful with anything that has that kind of power over us. For me, it's pizza.

# DEPRESSION

Depression is a fickle thing. Most of the time we can identify the cause. Other times depression seems to sneak up on us in spite of all the things going well in our world. If we start to notice symptoms of depression in our mood or outlook, one of the first things we need to do is survey the past couple of months.

In particular, look at the things you might file under the heading "stressful." Stressful things include (but aren't limited to) job changes, relationship changes, physical health decline, or injury. These are some pretty common stressful things in our lives that can greatly impact our mood. If you've experienced one or more of these changes, you might have just pinpointed a significant source of depression.

It's also not unusual for us to feel symptoms of depression in our bodies. An increase or decrease in appetite, for example, is a common physical expression of depression. We may find ourselves eating more than we typically do, later into the evening than we typically do, or eating for emotional reasons instead of hunger reasons. It's also not uncommon to start having difficulty sleeping. People with depression often find themselves waking up in the middle of the night and having difficulty going back to sleep. That leads to fatigue and low energy during the day.

When we're constantly stressed out, negative thoughts begin to creep in. We become harsh and critical of ourselves and of others. We misread things in our environment as negative when in fact they're either neutral or even positive. And when we misread things in our world as negative, it reflects on our internal state.

If activities in our lives just don't seem to be as pleasurable or as interesting as they used to be, keep an eye on the situation. If our moods continue in that direction, we're inclined to step away from activities that are good for our wellbeing and state of mind. When we do that, we increase the likelihood of isolation.

We have to put the effort in when it comes to keeping symptoms of depression at bay. That means we make the conscious decision to participate in the activity we once enjoyed, even if we're feeling depleted. It means we reach out to others, even when we don't feel like socializing.

Depression is surmountable, but it takes a willingness to do things we know are healthy for us, no matter what we're feeling in the moment.

# DESTRUCTION AWAITS THOSE WHO ISOLATE

Face it, sometimes our best thinking is terrible thinking. We believe we have our heads on straight, but bubbling underneath us are challenges that impact our judgment in ways we don't always realize.

We become our own saboteurs in the blink of an eye by making one big, irrational decision.

Good news is there are ways to save us from ourselves! One proven way is to run our decisions by trusted friends before we act on them. This is especially true when we find ourselves in life's valleys where we're struggling with something personal.

We all need to find someone who can be our sounding board, someone we share personal things with, someone who won't judge us. These are the people who have no problem looking us in the eye and sincerely asking, "Have you lost your (insert expletive) mind?"

For example, let's say we're stressed or feeling anxious, so we decide to go shopping. But this isn't going to be just any shopping spree—we're going binge-shopping. In fact, we're going to max out the credit card because lots of new things will make us feel better!

Or maybe we have a couple of kids and our spouse doesn't have a lot of time for us. So, we think to ourselves, "Hey, here's a good idea. I'll have an affair with my co-worker. That'll be fun, spontaneous, and if nobody finds out, won't destroy my marriage. Why didn't I think of this before?"

See how crazy these ideas sound when you read them? Now, imagine telling a trusted friend about your decision in a casual conversation over a latte at the coffee shop. That's why it's important to tell someone what's running through your head when you're struggling. What we need the most is a trusted friend, somebody who will step in and say, "Yeah, that's a terrible idea, don't do it!"

Of course, there are some rules of engagement to consider when sharing your great ideas with friends. First and foremost, give your confidant ALL of the information. This isn't the time to be shy. Let it all hang out—the good, the bad, and the ugly. I can't tell you how often I asked people if they told their friends all about their plans before they acted on them. It's extremely rare if they have, like chance-of-getting-hit-by-lightning rare.

So is it really any wonder why our friends give us "bad" advice when we give them "bad" or "incomplete" information? Don't do that! We'd be better off not saying anything to them. We may even run the risk of them thinking the idea is good.

We need voices of reason because we don't think clearly when we isolate. In fact, when we isolate, we listen only to the voices in our head—and we all know that some of those voices don't exactly give the best advice. When we give them consideration, some die right away while others will need more work. If we can rid ourselves of the worst ideas, the best path forward sometimes gets a little clearer.

If we're going to avoid self-sabotage, we really need other people listening to our thoughts, ideas, and struggles. In the stormiest times of life, we need to use our best thinking, which means we're actively seeking counsel from those we trust. Piece of advice: always get a piece of advice.

# FEAR

We're in uncharted territory.

Thanks to globalization and connectivity, we are more aware of the accidents, attacks, violence, and bad things that can happen in the world. They have crept into our living rooms, laptops, and mobile devices. Our community, which used to be fairly limited, has ballooned into a place where it can seem like violence happens every day. And, yes, violence happens every day in the world, but it's not true that violence happens every day in my community. And by community I mean my family, street, neighborhood, school, and office.

What's worse is that when violence and bad things do happen, we have an overabundance of information, videos, and images at our fingertips that exacerbate the problem. This can lead to fear and anxiety, which can cause us to act in ways that are simply out of character.

Exercising caution is never a bad idea. But, allowing fear to take control and prevent us from living well is something we have to guard against. Now more than ever.

It's important to remember that our outlook on life is largely predicated on a lifetime of thoughts, feelings, and experiences.

Most of our good decisions reflect a blend of these factors. Relying too much on any one of them leads to poor decision-making. In the case of anxiety, our thoughts, feelings, and experiences are exaggerated, and we often become catastrophic in our thinking, which leads us to greater levels of fear. It starts a cycle that increases and drives decisions that impact our relationships and lives.

We can start by consuming news responsibly. The twenty-four-hour news cycle and social media access can overload us with information that magnifies an event in our minds. When something horrible happens, we have almost immediate access to graphic pictures, iPhone videos, eyewitness accounts, and endless news stories. The more we watch an event, the more it settles into our mind's database. We have to limit how much we watch and take in and step away when we find ourselves obsessively reviewing the coverage.

When we find ourselves limiting our activities because of fear, we should pause to examine the reasoning behind our choices. If we don't take a more rational approach, we risk making our world so small that we miss out on life. We have to allow our rational thoughts to mix in with our emotional thoughts to form a realistic perspective on our safety and the probability of danger.

It's the same as not getting on an airplane. Even though flying is far safer than driving a car, irrational fear can easily consume us and negatively impact our lives.

The reality is that terrorist attacks, plane crashes, and other tragedies simply don't happen as often as we might think. The overload of information (and not just stories we heard from someone else, but the constant stream of videos and pictures we see) has led to a distortion in our view of the world. If we aren't careful, we can allow our thoughts to fill us with fear. Or, we can use them to help us navigate this uncharted territory with confidence and reason.

# DO YOU HAVE A DRINKING PROBLEM OR A PROBLEM WITH YOUR DRINKING?

Yeah, you may need to read that title again. It's important, or else I wouldn't ask you to. A small group of people have a drinking problem (addiction); a much bigger group of people consume alcohol in a way that causes problems in their life. Not an addiction, but a problem that may require assistance.

Why this discussion? Because I see individuals, couples, and families suffer unnecessarily. When we have problems in life, they often occur on a spectrum, from mild to moderate to severe. Whether we are talking about cholesterol, obesity, hair loss, or alcohol consumption, there is a range of illness and a range of treatment.

When it comes to alcohol, most people think that if you have had a mild or moderate problem, you need a high level of treatment. Something like Alcoholics Anonymous (AA) or residential treatment.

Well-respected physicians and providers in my field will sometimes say, "Yeah, you need to go to some meetings to treat the problems you're having with alcohol." But because those meetings are for people with more serious addictions, they're probably not for you if you're on the other end of the spectrum.

One of the reasons people who deal with disordered drinking don't get better is because they think that AA or an alcohol addiction treatment center are their only options. They are not.

You may be a mom who's been drinking a little too much wine with the other moms during those "Chardonnay play dates" or after the kids are in bed. You may be a husband who's come in drunk a few nights—not consistently, but enough that it has become a nuisance. In both cases, it's enough that you don't spend quite as much time with your spouse or kids. You probably don't need to go away, but you should definitely talk to somebody about what's going on.

I think AA does great work, but even AA will support my premise that it is for real alcoholics, not for those who drink more than they should now and again.

If you're dealing with a problem in your drinking and you see it impacting your family, your marriage, or those closest to you, you don't have to avoid getting help because AA and treatment centers don't seem right for you. In all likelihood, you need something a little different.

Instead, talk to somebody who has been working in the addiction field for some time who can talk to you about how you struggle. Find someone you can be accountable to who can help you look at the times and places and people that may influence how you drink.

I'm not saying you have a drinking problem, but can we agree that there have been a few times that your drinking has caused a problem? Okay then. Let's try to talk about how you would like to do things a little differently.

# WHEN THE WORST HAPPENS

A long-time friend recently opened up to me about an unimaginably painful time in his life. After years of working together, I was shocked to hear his tragic story of losing his child.

As we can all imagine, and as some of us can attest, losing a child is devastating. The emotional toll is immediate and deep.

My friend endured unspeakable loss, yet there he was telling me about this tragedy with strength and resilience. I had to ask him, "How did you make it through?"

I'll never forget his answer. "I just decided it was a chapter of my life, a horrible chapter," he said. "It's not going to be *the* chapter of my life."

I was struck by that perspective. It rang true. It is the kind of wisdom that is born out of great suffering. And in that short statement there are a few things to hang on to.

One is that we must recognize the short-term nature of tragedy. Sadness, despair, and hardship only last for a season. They don't last forever. Yes, it's an unbearable, difficult chapter in our lives, and we must find ways to be resilient, push ahead, and limit the experience to just one chapter of our lives. Too often we make it our book, and we may not have to.

For some who have endured tragedy, the season of pain and struggle becomes the defining season. It can define them in a way that is limiting to the rest of their lives. They become a diagnosis, a tragedy, or a victim. They allow bitterness, resentment, anger, and sadness to rise to such levels that it inhibits their ability to deal with pain and move on to the brighter seasons of life.

The other truth of his statement is that other seasons in life are coming. Things may get better, and unexpected blessings often come from tragedy.

When we find ourselves turning the last page of that difficult experience, we have to be mindful of how our emotions are influencing our next chapter. If we aren't careful, we will take some beliefs and feelings to the next chapter and the next and the next. Then we find ourselves wondering how we got to this place. Usually, it's one chapter at a time. We work through our horrible chapter in a way that helps prevent it from defining our whole existence.

There is more in life to experience. Even when the worst happens, the seasons of life never stop changing. Where winter leaves, spring picks things up. I know it's not easy, but it's possible.

And I think it is how we need to look at this story of ours, this life. Struggle well in that chapter, and then hope for—and work for—a chapter where you will live well.

# SUFFERING CAN HAVE HIDDEN BENEFITS

Before you get too far into this concept, realize that I'm not saying we should seek suffering or desire it so we can "grow." But let's be honest, it's a difficult world. There's no way around that fact. And in this often cruel world, we as human beings go through long and short stretches of suffering, whether we brought them on ourselves or fate decided it was our turn to play the punching bag.

Yes, suffering sucks. But what if I told you suffering can also bring growth and may even be necessary if we want to enrich our lives?

Sometimes we make the mistake of thinking it's our job to take away people's suffering. Whether you're a parent, counselor, pastor, or just a friend, your job is to give hope, encouragement, and support in the midst of suffering, not to make it all go away. No, I'm not saying we intentionally leave people in their suffering. Usually it has to run its course, and there is not much we can do to hurry it along. So, spend your energy in a place it can bear fruit. Sit, have a meal, or go for a walk with someone in a difficult time. Relationships are healing.

Suffering can also be the road to insight. Suffering sometimes forces us to slow down, to eliminate things from our daily routine, and to create a space to reflect. Difficult times can bring strength and the confidence to make it through challenges. As we meet these challenges, we begin to believe in our own strength and in our ability to lean on the strength of friends.

If you're a parent and you continue to be the genie in your kids' lives who makes all their problems go away, you will deprive them of the life experiences they need to learn, grow, and mature into functional, well-rounded adults. Our ability to tolerate our children's difficulties is directly related to their ability to grow. If it's "too much for us," they won't learn what life is trying to teach.

Suffering also amplifies the bright spots in life. It allows us to better appreciate the beauty and wonder that this world has to offer, in spite of all the hardships we might be facing. We can find gratitude for things that we didn't even notice the day before. We can be reminded of the gifts in our life, the ways we have been blessed, and the connection we have with others who suffer.

Lastly, the endurance of great suffering has come to define the power of the human spirit. People like Holocaust survivor Viktor Frankl who went on to become an icon of humanity's resilience in the face of adversity. There are great examples of this concept with people and situations through the ages. If they can find meaning and purpose and strength in such dire circumstances, then it gives me hope for my own situation. And by the way, how they dealt with suffering also gave strength and hope to those close to them. Sometimes that's the most important thing that comes from our struggles.

Yes, this world is often cruel, but it is full of awe and wonder as well. If we're able to open our eyes in the midst of our suffering or be present when others are suffering, we might be able to see how inspiring our world really is.

# CHAPTER
## eight
# SERENITY

# REALLY? YOU THINK YOU CONTROL THAT?

Take a second to answer this: How much of your world do you control? By control I mean determine, dictate, and decide what other people do. What percentage?

My answer? Less than ten percent!

Stay with me here.

We don't control nearly as much as we think we do and that fundamentally shifts our expectations. When we think we can control people and situations, we dwell on what we can't change rather than what's within our control. We tighten our grip so fervently that our hands cramp and go numb. That's when our circumstances slip through our fingers. And how does that make us feel? Yeah, frustrated. Angry. Sad. Possibly even vengeful.

What's the natural reaction to these emotions? We overcorrect to the point of being wrong again.

Such is the conundrum of control: the more we try to control, the more out of control we feel. Suddenly, all of the order we've tried to create turns to organized chaos.

Even thinking about taking control can lead us to obsess over all the things that we perceive to be broken. We start doing all kinds of things to ensure the outcome, coordinating and moving heaven and earth so that things work out the way we want them to. Or, more accurately, like we need them to. Ultimately, we're haunted by what's missing or wrong and look past what's whole and life-affirming. And that can be the road to, well, Hell.

Which brings to mind one of my favorite quotes, the *Serenity Prayer* by Reinhold Niebuhr: "God, grant me the serenity to accept the things I cannot change, courage to change the things I can, and the wisdom to know the difference."

The Serenity Prayer was used to inject some much-needed hope and perspective into the lives of people who struggle. Alcoholics Anonymous has since adopted and adapted the prayer to use with those suffering from alcoholism. The prayer is a tool to approach life, not just a particular obstacle. That's how it has become so well known and well used.

There are aspects of our lives that we can change; our thoughts, lifestyle choices, and relationships with loved ones. These are elements of our lives that we should try to change for the better. And when it comes to the things we can't change—such as other people's actions, the past, or the future—we need to learn to acknowledge them and then move on. We need to candidly accept that there are things that we can't change. Then we have to stay alert so that we don't slip back into the role of changer. Do we want to be happy or do we want to be right? Often, we can't have both, especially if we're married. *Are we going to be better, or are we going to be bitter?*

The greatest act of control that we could demonstrate is to admit we don't have the level of control we think we do. Once we accept that realization, our lives will start to feel lighter, a tad bit easier, and all those thoughts racing through our head might just get a little quieter.

# WARNING: LABELS CAN BE HAZARDOUS TO YOUR HEALTH

"**S**o, tell me about yourself."

This seemingly benign request can often have a poisonous bite. Because like it or not, no matter what answer you give, no matter what words you use, a picture of you is going to get set in other people's minds.

We're a culture that likes to use labels. We like to paint people in broad strokes and then—*voila!*—call them complete. Assumption is our filler, and it's enough to make anyone trigger-shy when it comes to divulging even the most basic facts about themselves.

You tell people that you have depression? You've just become the "depressed guy," and nothing else about you seems to matter. In their eyes, you don't just *have* the illness; you *become* the illness.

You're a Christian? No worries, your opinions and moral principles are already declared for you by strangers—by people who think they know everything about you because they know that one single thing.

Though we might try to use labels to deepen our understanding of others, what we usually end up with are misconceptions about the person.

Some of this is caused by how politicized labels have become. The media warps the narrative so that entire communities become defined by a single issue or a cluster of presuppositions. Test yourself on these terms: LGBT rights. Hispanics. Muslims. White people.

Any thoughts or feelings come to mind? For all of the openness and conversations we claim to have, we seem to be drawing more lines among ourselves than ever. We are eliminating the thing that fosters connections between people. When we label human beings, we inevitably turn them into something less than human. We lose the individual because of the group.

If we were to make an honest effort to have meaningful discussions about identities and beliefs, we might find ourselves in a world that is far more caring and compassionate than the system we have now.

# EXPECT RESISTANCE FROM YOURSELF

Resisting new things is a normal part of changing behavior. We're creatures of habit, plain and simple. But we can also make some amazing changes and embark on new paths. We *can* change.

No matter how much we tell ourselves that change is good for us, it still feels *uncomfortable*. I was working with a swim coach who told me to swim one length of the pool. I did, and then he told me what I was doing wrong with my right elbow (I still don't know how he could see that kind of detail). He told me what to do and then to swim down and back again. I did. He asked how it felt, and I quickly replied, "Awkward. I felt like a shark attack victim; surprised I didn't drown." He laughed and said it looked perfect.

It doesn't matter if it's swimming, eating better, or starting to manage our emotions better—"new" always feels a little awkward. It doesn't mean it's wrong, just different. And that's completely natural. In fact, it's often the best way to tell that we're headed in the right direction. And it's almost enough to make us want to quit and fall back into our old patterns. But stay with it; it will become your new normal.

The trick is to embrace the discomfort, see it as normal. When we do, we start to lose the need to get away from it. We feel and think differently. If we do that, we might start to experience the situation differently and see things that we had been missing.

It's a game of pros and cons. We look at the disadvantages of our current behavior and the advantages of behaving differently. We look at it in terms of what we stand to gain by altering our behavior instead of what we're giving up.

Frame it in terms of, *If I quit doing this, I might have more energy for this activity,* or, *If I quit doing this, then my relationship with my husband or wife might get better.*

When you weigh what you want against what you're doing to prevent yourself from getting it, you'll find that it's easy to find *your* reason to make a change.

In the short term, it might seem like punishment to push yourself into an uncomfortable situation or behavior, but in the long run, you'll find a new normal.

# BIASED, MOSTLY NEGATIVE?

When I was in grad school, a professor of mine always said, "You're all the good you say you are and all the bad you say you're not."

And I think that's exactly right.

We are very good at criticism. And part of that is just how our brains are wired. We have this thing called negative bias. It's a defense mechanism. But sometimes, we take that to an extreme. Part of it has to do with our external influences, and part of it has to do with our internal worlds. We take the guilt, the anxiety, the anger, and all of the other negative emotions we have, and we turn them in on ourselves.

It can become a commentary in our brains that runs on a constant loop: *You're not smart enough. You're not pretty enough. Nothing you say is interesting or insightful. Nothing you do is good enough. You always fall short.*

"We need a healthy dose of humility," you might be tempted to say. But, honestly, at a certain point, criticism becomes destructive. It can paralyze us from doing or saying what needs to be done or said. That's when we need to start looking for the good, for all of the things that we tell ourselves aren't there.

We need to find a way to fill in all of the holes we've poked in our self-confidence before we start to sink.

And maybe the easiest way to start that is to look at the people in your life and point out the things you admire about them: their kindness, their sense of humor, their willingness to help. You have to ask yourself what it is about other people that draws you in, and then you have to find those things in yourself.

They're there; I promise you.

Embrace those good things, and remind yourself that those are the things that everyone around you already sees.

Confidence in yourself comes from honesty with yourself. You have to own all of your shortcomings and faults, but you also have to counter every one of those with a virtue.

# THE GIFT OF A LIFETIME: LIVING IN THE PRESENT

The idea of living in the present, or living in the now, is not a new concept. In fact, it's been discussed so much that it has started taking on near mythic proportions. When we talk about this concept, it is always from the standpoint that what we are doing is robbing us of the joy we should have today. When we aren't enjoying today, it's not because we are remembering wonderful, joyful times or thinking about how wonderful things will be in the future.

What we tend to do when we struggle is focus on the negative, the painful or potentially painful things. We think that by doing that we are going to protect ourselves from hurt, from the dreaded phone call at 2:00 in the morning. To many of us, living in the present can seem like an impossibility.

If you are shaped by your past and constantly planning for your future, your present gets buried. Almost like it's not a real state of being at all. When today is burdened with the past and the future, the emotion is almost always fear or sadness. And that feeling leads to thoughts that are not going to help us be successful today.

We are afraid of making the same mistakes that we made in our past, and we are terrified that we are going to do something to jeopardize our future. That is a miserable, anxiety-ridden way to live. There is no fulfillment in that, no possible way of achieving happiness.

When we're not living in the present, we're not living our lives.

*Living* is a today thing, not a yesterday thing. When we're looking back or looking ahead too often, we are being passive and allowing our unchangeable pasts and our hypothetical futures to hold us hostage.

So, how do we re-center ourselves? How do we find a way to actually exist in our bodies, right here in the present moment?

Energy.

We have to project all of our energy, all of our focus, and all of our interest into the people we are with *right now*, the places we are *right now*, the things we are doing *right now*. Can you get lost in the conversation, in the movie, in the time on the beach and forget about all the other things? That's where we need to head, guarding those moments.

By doing that, we are becoming active participants in our lives, and we're doing it without having to think too hard about it. If we can engage in our present lives, it becomes easier to keep living that way; it becomes second nature.

Just like that, our past becomes more of a colorful album of memories than a series of fear-driven decisions, and our future becomes a bright, promising horizon of potential instead of a demanding, insurmountable wall.

We are never going to get rid of the uncertainty in our lives, but we don't have to add to the uncertainty by sitting stagnant and waiting for life to roll over us. We can take a role in shaping how it unfolds, always living with purpose and promise. That's what living in the moment is all about.

# BE QUIET

Recently, my wife and I went on vacation to one of our favorite beaches. It was our time to just lie on the beach and relax. But this time, I couldn't sit still. I couldn't relax. I was literally working at trying to enjoy the beauty of the beach, the time with my wife, and the fact that I didn't have any work to do. I thought my unrest would settle by the end of the first day. It didn't. So, I settled in knowing for sure I'd be able to "relax" sometime that second day. Still no. I just continued to turn over all the things I needed to do, places I needed to go, people I needed to talk with. I simply couldn't slow my mind. I had to work to get to that place of enjoying the moment. It wasn't until the third day that I was able to settle my mind.

The struggle to relax and enjoy the day was a fantastic reminder of the need we have to be still, to just be quiet. One of the burdens of technology is that we have a constant ability to entertain ourselves with music, information, and family. And yes, it has some perks. But I see more downside than I do benefits. You can save up all your vacation time, spend your reward or mileage points, and go a couple thousand miles away only to discover you packed all the troubles and hassles of work and family in your luggage.

We actually talk quite a bit about this concept of being quiet. Our minds are running faster than they ever have. We are sorting more information and more data than our forefathers could have imagined. And all that activity comes at a price.

I think that's where meditation comes in. We do better when we settle ourselves and have a little bit of time away from all of the noise and our thoughts. It gives our minds and our bodies a time to recharge. I don't think it matters if we do it every day, a couple of times a week, or once a month. But

I definitely think it matters. When we find ourselves struggling, it means we need to do something different or learn a new skill. Like being quiet and at rest both in our mind as much as in our body.

I hate learning lessons on vacation. But, boy, did I feel better from day three on.

# ENLIGHTENED

# DON'T BE AN ASS

This entry title is actually the best piece of advice I have ever heard given to graduate students. It came from a tenured professor and is his very succinct advice for students as they begin to venture out into "the real world" and begin working for other people. Genius!

To be fair, we all have certain times or difficult seasons where we *act* like an ass. Not unusual, and most of the time we apologize for our behavior or attitude. We are even aware of when we act this way—when we treat people like they aren't important or when we get so absorbed in our own desires that we walk right over our friends. We know it and respond appropriately, apologizing.

The professor's caution was for people like that, good people who get stressed by deadlines, feel the pressure of performance, think their ideas are the best because they had great grades in college, or want to meet the expectations of people they love. All those things are good, but taken to an inappropriate level, they can lead good people to act, well, like an ass. And good people, the kind of people you want in your life to make you a better person, don't like people like that. They're not good prospects for friendship.

When we step into the world of work, we quickly realize that we don't take any exams, don't write any papers, and don't get to have the fastest time in the race. Our success in the office and in life is more about our social understanding, our ability to navigate the unwritten rules and guidelines of life. People choose who they want to be with. Nobody chooses somebody that's an ass. We have to be good coworkers, good friends, good roommates. After school, nobody is forced to be with you in class or on the team. People choose who they want to be with. Nobody chooses somebody that's an ass.

So what do you do? Pursue a path that includes people you trust who can let you know when you're oblivious to how other people think about you. We need to avoid people who tell us what they think we want to hear, and we need to avoid people who have *the* right answer for our problem before we have even explained all the issues. We need people in the middle, people who will tell us the truth and ask good questions. These people know us well enough and care about us enough to deliver a difficult message. And telling a good friend that they acted like an ass is a difficult conversation. You only do it with people you care about. Or the guy who cut you off in traffic and will never see you again.

Now, there is another kind of person who acts like an ass seven days a week. It's become their way of interacting in the world, with their friends, and in the office. Sometimes they are really successful, usually lonely, but their success doesn't include others. These people? Avoid them. I do.

# DON'T TRY TO MAKE A VALID POINT BETTER

When we have a valid point, we should make it, then walk away. Don't walk away from the person or the conversation; just walk away from saying more about it. The minute we attempt to add to our point, we reduce its initial impact. In fact, ongoing petitions to prove our point only invite skepticism, or possibly rejection entirely. (Of course, if our intent is to just be rude and hurtful, then yeah, let's keep yammering on.)

Here are a couple of surefire ways we devalue our point. (Hint: let's avoid them!)

We'll call the first one, *strength in numbers*. This is when we reference other people who we think share our perceptions and support our position. Because if more people believe it, our point must be *more* true, right? It's like we're saying, "Hey, it's not just me! Ralph and Curt think like this, too!"

Let's be honest though; how often does that work? Short answer is never. In fact, pulling someone else into the conversation distracts from our initial valid point. And most often, the experiences we have with other people and situations are limited. We should focus our discussion on what we saw, heard, and felt. Keep our concerns to our observations and force the discussion of our thoughts and beliefs. (Side note: let's also be aware that our perceptions aren't always accurate.)

A second way we decrease the heaviness of a valid point is when we get historical. This is the classic version of including as many situations, statements, or scenarios from the past that support our valid point. If your spouse shares something at dinner with friends that you feel was embarrassing, talk about that dinner with her and what she said that night, once you are in the car or at home. Don't relive and rehash the discussion by talking about the dinner with family at Thanksgiving, breakfast with your old roommate, and the guy at the health club as further examples of how she "always" does this.

By footnoting our point with past events, we admit that our valid point is weak and needs supporting evidence. I get why we do it. But, it rarely works. Valid points are specific to a situation, conversation, or person. When we generalize it, it feels like somebody's trying to make a bigger statement. It's normal to feel a little startled or caught off guard when somebody challenges us with something that is personal, something that we know but may not be ready to admit.

So if you have a valid point, help make it a little easier for that person and keep your point small, short, succinct. You're saying something to somebody that they don't see. That's hard to receive. Let them drink their glass of water. No need to put a fire hose down their throat.

Another way we devalue our point is actually one of my favorites. I call it the *presentation of absolute certainty*. When we present our valid point as though it's a fact, we weaken our position. Our perceptions are never that certain, and they aren't that certain because we bring a host of expectations, fears, dreams, and hurts to life. We don't need to act with such absolute certainty when we have a valid point. People who have valid points have a calm presentation. It's unshakeable in a quiet way.

If you can articulate  a clear, precise thought and succinctly communicate your point-of-view, then you've done your job. Now hold it. Let it sit. Let it breathe.

# WHAT WILL I BE WHEN I GROW UP?

**W**e're asked that question all our lives, and depending on our age, we come up with different answers. As kindergarteners, we color "what we want to be when we grow up" on activity sheets. As high school students, we daydream about careers to get us through homework or even pen essays about careers as part of our homework. As college students, we break into a cold sweat when we hear this question (especially from our parents) and avoid giving answers.

Recently, somebody asked me what I anticipated as the "next steps" in my career. I laughed and replied, "I'm not sure what I want to be when I grow up." And I was kind of serious. It was a wonderful older gentleman who, at the end of a very successful career and life, presented the right question at the right time in my life. We were talking about one of his children when he said, "It doesn't matter what you do for a living. It matters who you are."

Yes! That's what matters. Ask anybody over the age of forty and they'll likely respond the same way. Our careers are a lot less important than who we are. We probably have the talent to do a number of things really well. But, is that what we want to define us? I've never seen a tombstone that said anything about being an accountant, lawyer, welder, electrician, or nurse.

If we're not sure what exactly does define us, we should honestly ask ourselves, "What are we most proud of in our lives?" If the answer is only about what we do for a living, it may be time to do some more thinking. Don't get me wrong; we should be proud of what we do and how we do it. But is that what we want to be known for? I think we want more.

No matter what shape our answers take—be it our inner child's desire to fly on a unicorn or drive a firetruck, our teenage dream of being rich and famous, or just a desire to find a job after college—it's a fascinating question. But, it's not necessarily the best one.

141

I believe one of our greatest challenges with that question is that it highlights our emphasis on the wrong things. We're influenced by family, friends, and society to construct our future based on a particular career path. Our self-worth then becomes dependent on what our career will or won't do for us.

Of course, we need jobs and careers. They're critical to providing for our needs and supplementing our wants. But, we have to guard against our career becoming more than it really is. If you pay attention to people who have achieved "success," almost all of them respond the same way when asked about their career success. They don't talk about the career; they talk about the personal elements of the career. They talk about the kind of person they have become and how others feel about them as a person.

Creating a perfect vision of who we want to become and what we will be remembered for can start now, regardless of the direction we're currently going in life.

*Where* do I want to be? *Who* do I want to be? Now those are questions worth pondering.

# WHEN AND WHERE

My kids have heard this mantra much of their lives; in fact, they still do. I used it a lot when they were young and wanted to try their hand at being funny. It usually sounded something like "Did you really think that was the best time to say that to your mother?" or "Do you really think that you should have tried that in the back seat of the car?" When and Where.

Seeing they seemed to understand that little guidance, I have continued to use the questions as they have mastered their humor and now turn their attention to mastering the art of living well. The art of knowing when to step off the well-trodden path of life and when to stay on it.

To be clear, the well-worn path is a good path—it's comfortable, secure, predictable, and there are many people on it. And it can help us at times when we struggle. Now, there are times we decide to do something great, daring to step on some new unbroken path. And that's when life can get interesting.

We all know people who would never even dream of stepping off the path and those that can't even seem to find the path with a flashlight. I'm not really talking about people like that.

I'm talking about those who have a desire and feel a call to try something they think and feel deeply about. Individuals who struggle with a decision because they feel two ways about a subject, creating an inner turmoil that begs to be resolved.

Embrace that feeling. Yes, it is terrible and exhilarating all at the same time. When you're there, it means you are thinking about doing something great in your life—something you have talked with others about, dreamed about, and maybe even penciled the plans of on a napkin. Stay with that discomfort until it pulls you forward.

And at moments like that, guard against fear, worry, and what it would mean if things went incredibly bad. That will not steady your nerves or focus your thoughts.

And when people say "be careful," just know they really mean "that scares me."

It can make people nervous to see others walking on a different path. Parents get nervous when their kids want to pursue a degree in the arts instead of business or when, heaven forbid, they decide to strike out on their own sans college or pursue the "alternate career path."

If you've got a flame inside of you that standard operating procedure just can't extinguish, then it's time to break the rules. Be the exception. Take the leap. Just be sure to make a plan before you jump. And start forging an iron stomach now. You're going to need it.

It takes a lot of courage to make a new path. Because even with an extraordinary talent and a clear personal vision, you can still fail. But, that life lesson is a reward in its own right. It's the bump in the road on the way to where many have found greatness.

# A GOOD BOOK IS BETTER THAN A BAD THERAPIST

True statement. You may be shocked that a study or two found it to be true as well.

We think too narrowly about the definition of therapy. We sometimes say, "That was therapeutic," after a wickedly difficult cycling class or trip to the gym. And that's the effect good books have on us. They can be amazingly therapeutic.

Now, I'm not talking about a self-help book. Although I don't mind them and have even used them myself. I'm talking about a book with a story and characters we can become invested in. The kind of book that gives us a world to fall into and lose ourselves for a while. A place to explore and wonder.

Reading enables us to loosen an emotional valve and gives us a chance to widen our introspective scope. And when we do that a funny thing can happen. We can find ourselves thinking about things and perspectives that we hadn't considered.

Books can even give us the distance we sometimes need to explore an issue. Sometimes, issues are too close to the surface for us to talk about with friends or family. But a good book can sneak up on us when our defenses are resting. And that's when good stuff happens.

Reading about characters in stories allows us to connect with them, see their struggles, and find the ones we can identify with. What does that mean? It's basically a big "me too" vote of support for the character, and we get to ride along and see how someone else sees our struggle, how they navigate their world carrying the same load we carry. What do they think, what do they feel, how do they manage their life, and what surprises us about how they do it? And if we can allow ourselves to ride along, defenses down, we might just walk away a different person.

Great books can also help us heal. Viktor Frankl's *Man's Search for Meaning* is one of those books. As a Holocaust survivor, Frankl witnessed the worst side of humanity. Yet, in his book, he reinforces the idea that meaning can be found in any circumstance, even in the midst of suffering. And perhaps most encouraging is the message that those who experience horrible events in life can go on to lead meaningful and joyful lives. Sometimes we need other people to give words to our suffering, validate its importance, and breathe hope into our lives.

In books, we can find truths that we have yet to see in ourselves, discover language for things we don't even know we're feeling, and learn to engage with our feelings in a healthy way.

The art of reading is essential. Get lost in it and see what you find. It's an art we can't afford to lose.

# WHAT TRIBE ARE YOU IN?

It doesn't matter who we are. We need a tribe. Whether we're a socialite, introvert, extrovert, educated, salt of the earth…we need a tribe. We need a small circle of people who know us as well as we know them. We need to know and be known. Maybe we have one or two members in our tribe already. That's a start! But let's try and make it three to five.

We refer to them in different ways—my girls, my buddies, my family, my tribe, or my people. We're talking about that small group we know is important because life is difficult. We're going to struggle. And when we struggle, people are the most significant source of healing in our lives. If I've learned anything over the past several decades of working with people during their struggles, it's the value of relationships. Like it or not, they're critical. We know from our experiences—and research just happens to confirm it—that meaningful relationships support healing and mental health and give us joy in our lives when we're struggling.

But if we're going to be in a tribe, we're going to have to invest in it. We're going to have to give up some time, energy, emotions, thoughts, and prayers; and we're going to have to be connected in a relational way. Yeah, it can be a hassle. It's sometimes messy, and it's not as fun as going on a long bike ride by yourself (I'm just saying). But the good news is that messy means growth. Hassle means healing.

Relationships don't usually develop in the midst of battle. It's in the midst of battle that we see what kind of relationships we've already developed. And we definitely don't want to find out we're lacking in trusted friends when we're pinned down in the trenches. Even if we have no one in our life and aren't all that concerned about it, we need to find somebody because we are going to struggle.

There are lots of places to find a tribe. Whether it's a neighbor, coworker, fellow student, yoga buddy, or group of people who share a similar hobby or passion for work, we should strive with all our might to get those people into our life. Friends do many of the same kinds of things that a clergy member, a therapist, or a support group do. And, to have them, we need to be ready to sacrifice some of our own time and effort. Healthy relationships are not one-way streets.

Life is difficult. We will struggle. But if we want to live well, we absolutely, positively need a tribe.

And if you happen to be seeing a therapist or psychiatrist at the moment, do me a favor: help them out a little. Get a tribe.

# EPILOGUE

I wrote this book to share what I've learned walking alongside people during the darkest chapters of their lives—some of the most amazing men and women, who were willing to struggle well in the pursuit of living well. And to share how I have walked through those hard chapters of my life as well. As many of you know, being present to these stories is a privilege that has a price. A price much higher than I ever realized.

And because of that, I have felt a greater need to share the things I, and the countless people like me whom I have been blessed to work alongside, have learned from these stories, these lives. It's in the sharing of stories that we see that our struggles can be used in ways that give us hope and encouragement.

I still wonder if I, Kevin, have anything worth sharing. "My" wisdom about life sounds like an odd concept. However, I have not a doubt that together we have a lot to share. And when I say "we," I mean all of us who have struggled to find better ways of dealing with the hard chapters because we believe that life shouldn't be this difficult, this painful, this challenging. Now that wisdom—the wisdom and lessons that I've learned from all those who have shared these experiences—"our" wisdom is a story I deeply believe is worth sharing as we learn to live well.

# ACKNOWLEDGEMENTS

*Struggle Well, Live Well* is the product of a lifetime journey—first to listen to others and then to figure out how best to say what I wanted to get across without sounding like a fool or embarrassing my loved ones. I'm not sure I accomplished either goal, but I can tell you that none of it would have been possible without the persistence and resilience of those who have allowed me or invited me to walk with them in a season of struggle.

Most importantly, I am grateful to my family, who makes my life (and its struggles) richer, fuller, and more complete than any one person deserves. Thank you Ann, Jennifer, Luke, and Lance. I would not be who I am, where I am, or where I am going without your help and patience. Truly.

I would like to thank a few decades worth of graduate students, clients, and coworkers who have been on this journey with me, especially my colleagues at Innovation360.

And, I'm immensely grateful for Team Kevin—Chris Kelley, Maureen Paulsen, and McGuire Boles of MPD Ventures Company; Aaron Cook; Danielle Fermier; Cindy Brown; the Maybell Group; and Bright Sky Press—who worked with me to make this book a reality.

Yes, it took a village to get this story told.

# BIOGRAPHY

Kevin Gilliland, Psy.D., is a licensed clinical psychologist and the Executive Director of Innovation360 (i360), an outpatient counseling service that works with people struggling with mental health, substance abuse, and relationship issues. Over the past twenty years, Kevin has mentored countless individuals and couples, participated in research trials, and lectured across the country. He currently serves in the Department of Dispute Resolution & Counseling at Southern Methodist University in Dallas where he instructs graduate students of the Annette Caldwell Simmons School of Education & Human Development. Outside of work, Kevin is an athlete and outdoorsman.

He regularly competes in triathlons and is a two time IRONMAN®. He and his wife, Ann, have three children—Jennifer, Luke, and Lance. They reside in Dallas, Texas.